Color By Number
For Beginners

Cover & Book Design by Nerine Martin
www.ColorYourWayToHappy.com

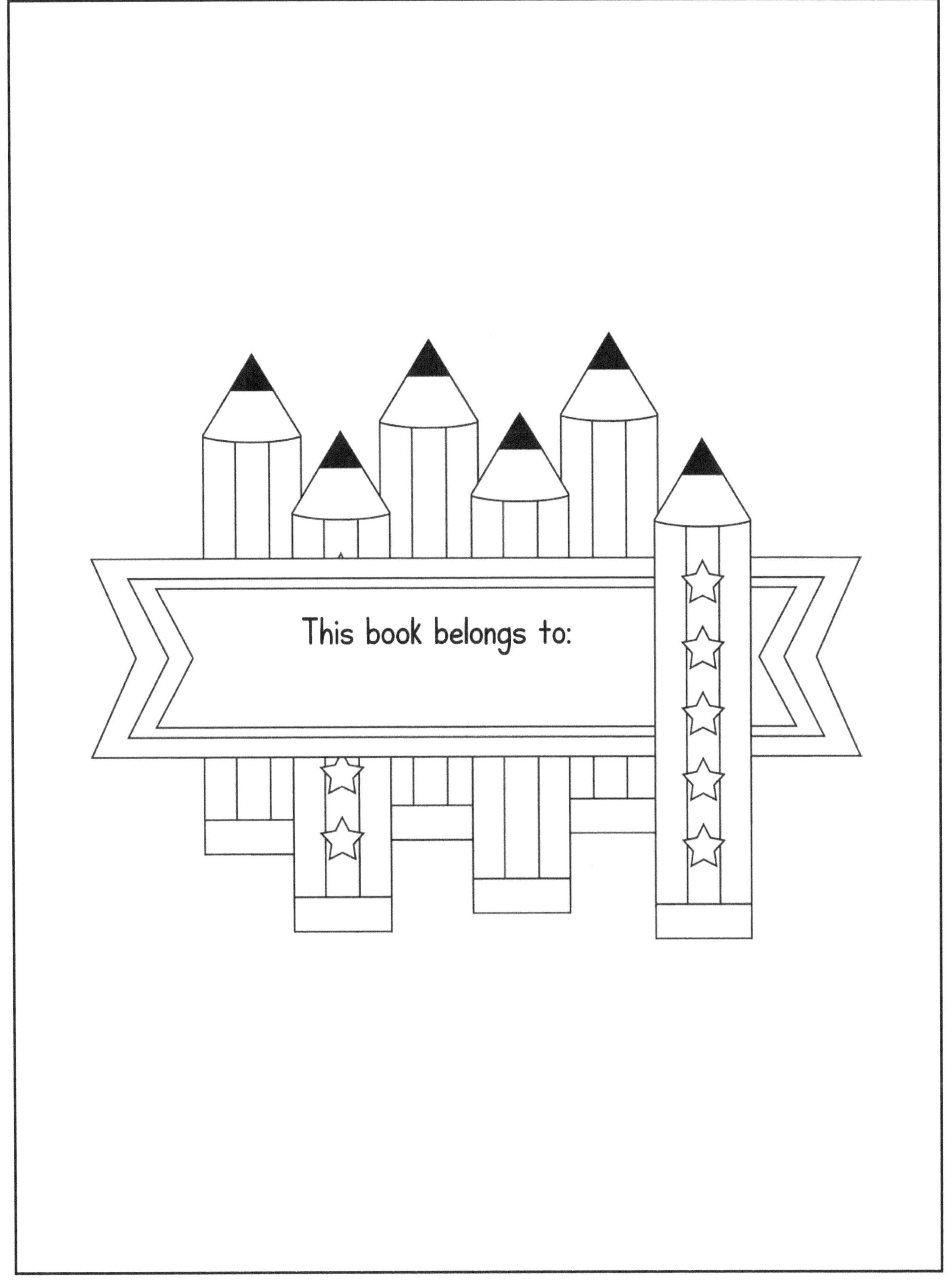

This book belongs to:

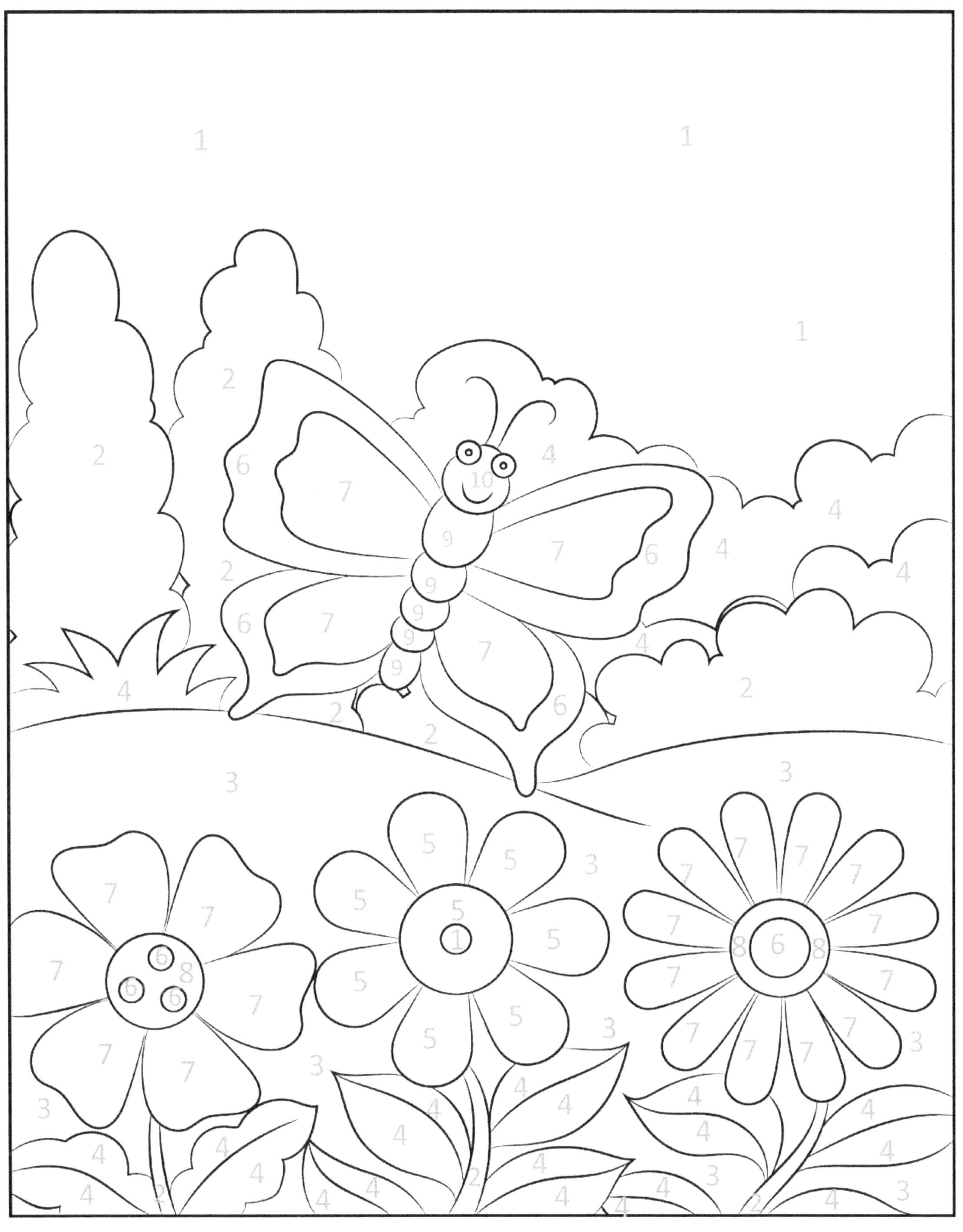

1 – Light Blue   3 – Light Green   5 – Blue   7 – Pink   9 – Black
2 – Green   4 – Dark Green   6 – Dark Pink   8 – Yellow   10 – Red

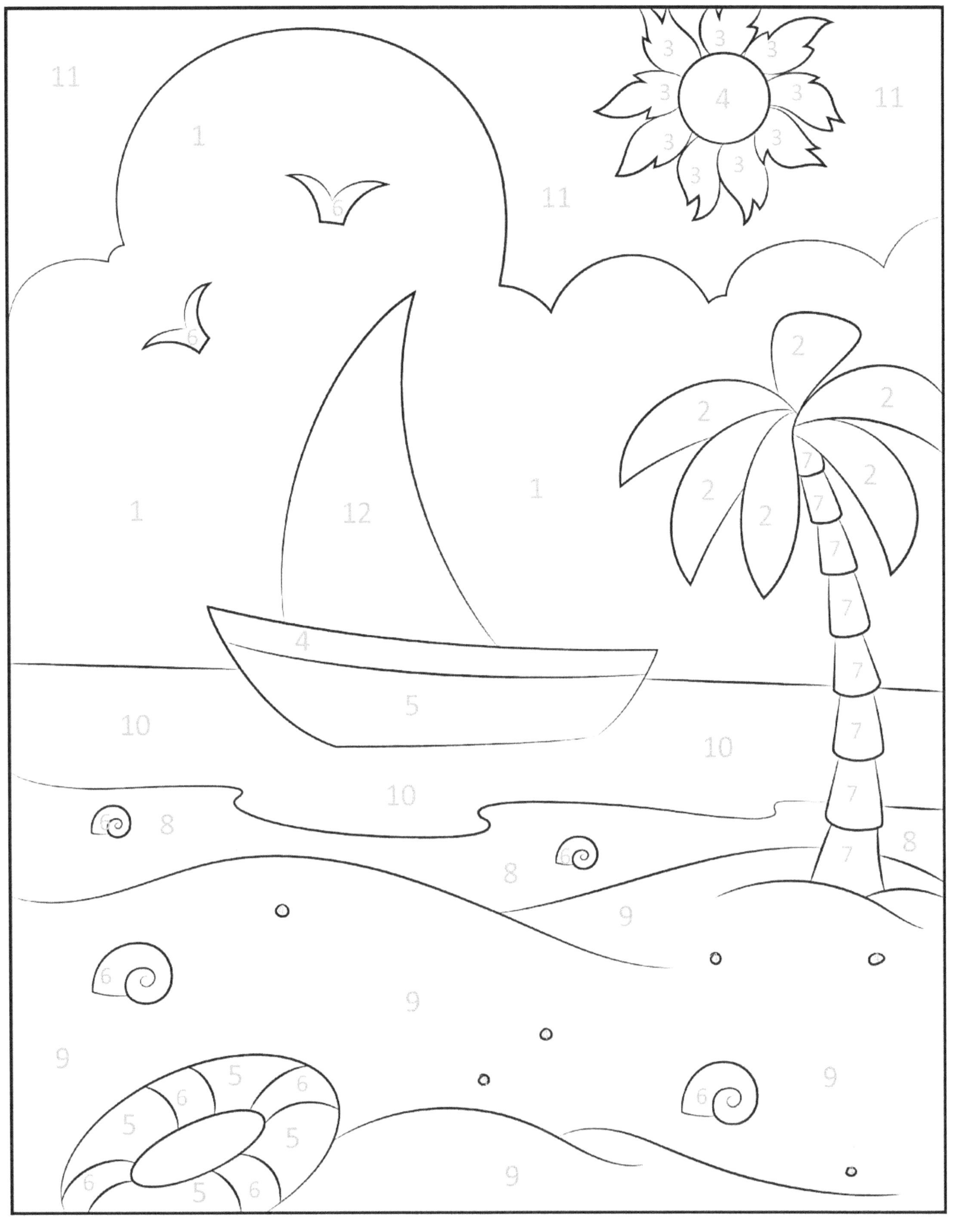

1 – Light Blue   3 – Yellow   5 – Red   7 – Dark Brown   9 – Light Yellow   11 – Blue
2 – Green   4 – Orange   6 – White   8 – Light Orange   10 - Dark Blue   12 - Purple

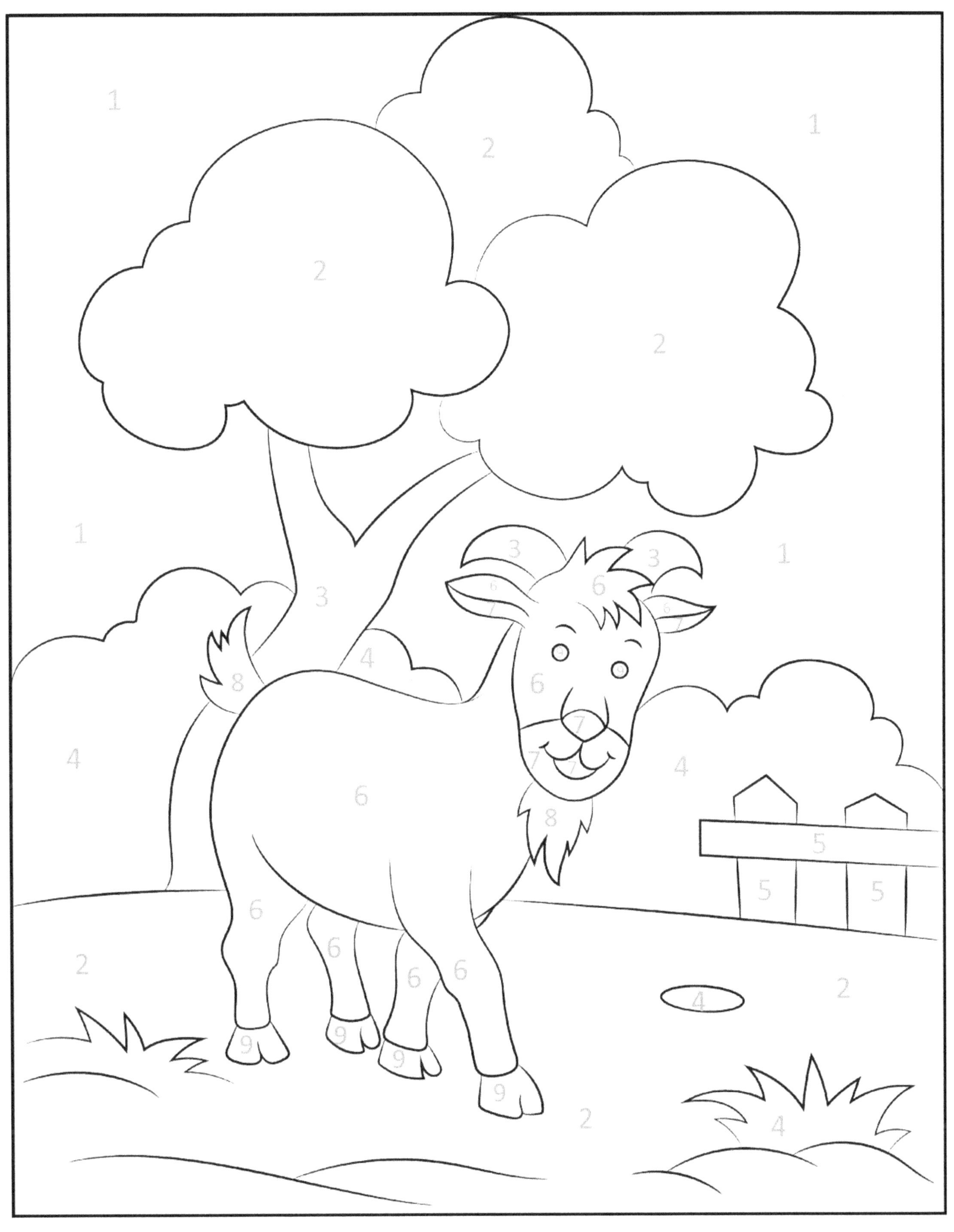

1 – Blue
2 – Green
3 – Brown
4 – Dark Green
5 – Orange
6 – White
7 – Pink
8 – Grey
9 – Black

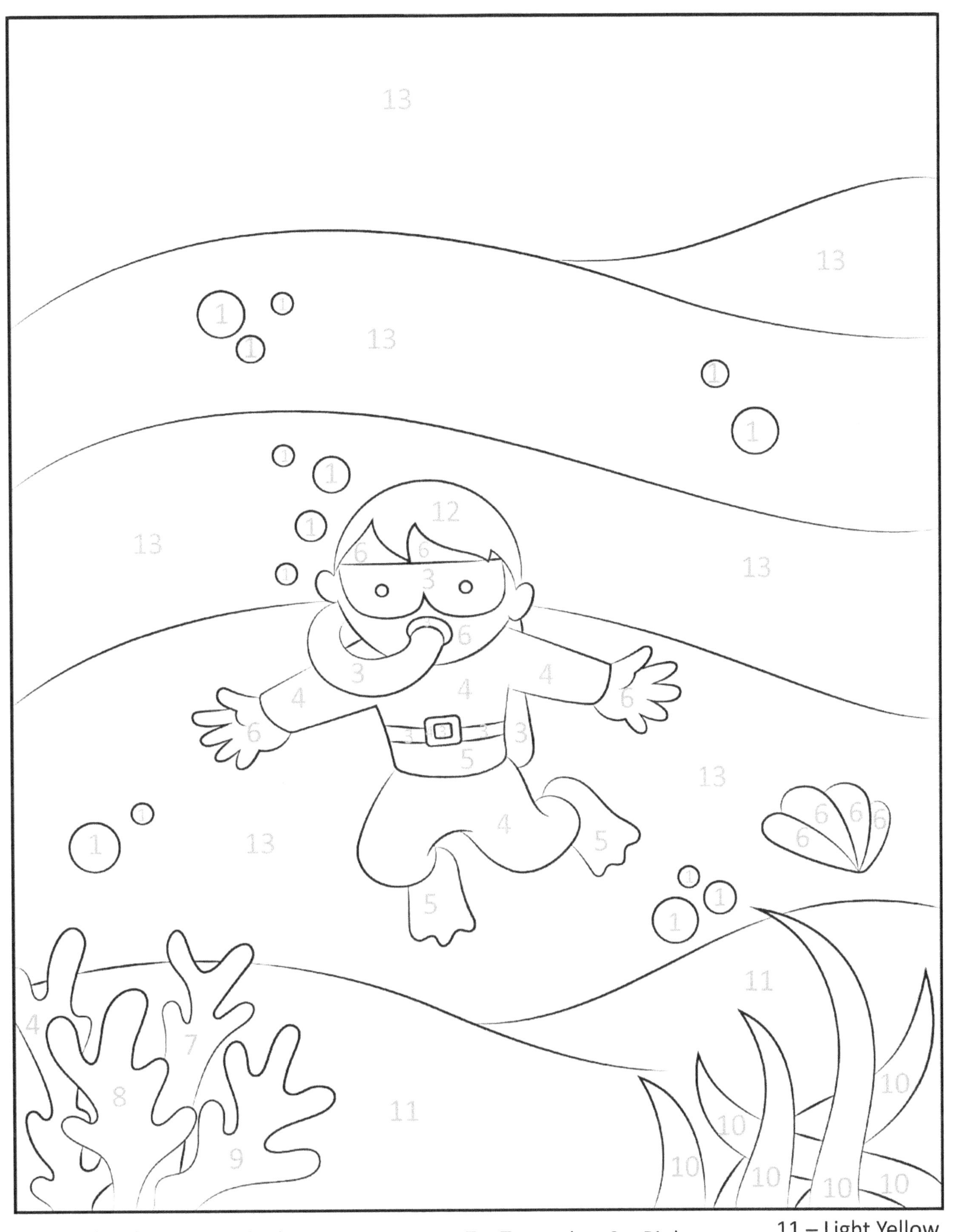

1 – Light Blue 3 – Dark Blue 5 – Orange 7 – Turquoise 9 – Pink 11 – Light Yellow
2 – White 4 – Yellow 6 – Light Pink 8 – Green 10 – Dark Green 12 – Brown
13 – Blue

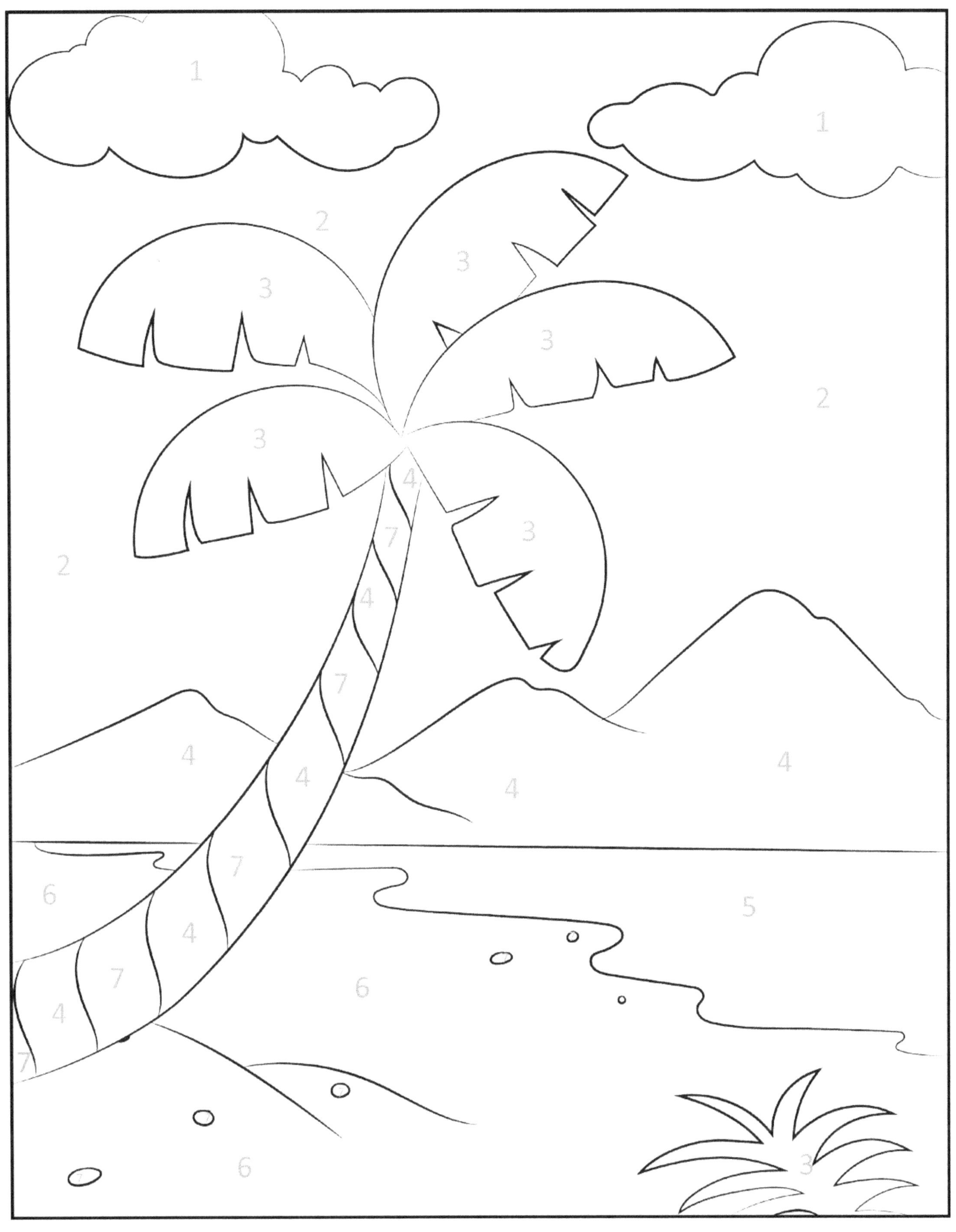

1 – Light Blue   3 – Green   5 – Turquoise   7 – Dark Brown
2 – Blue   4 – Brown   6 – Yellow

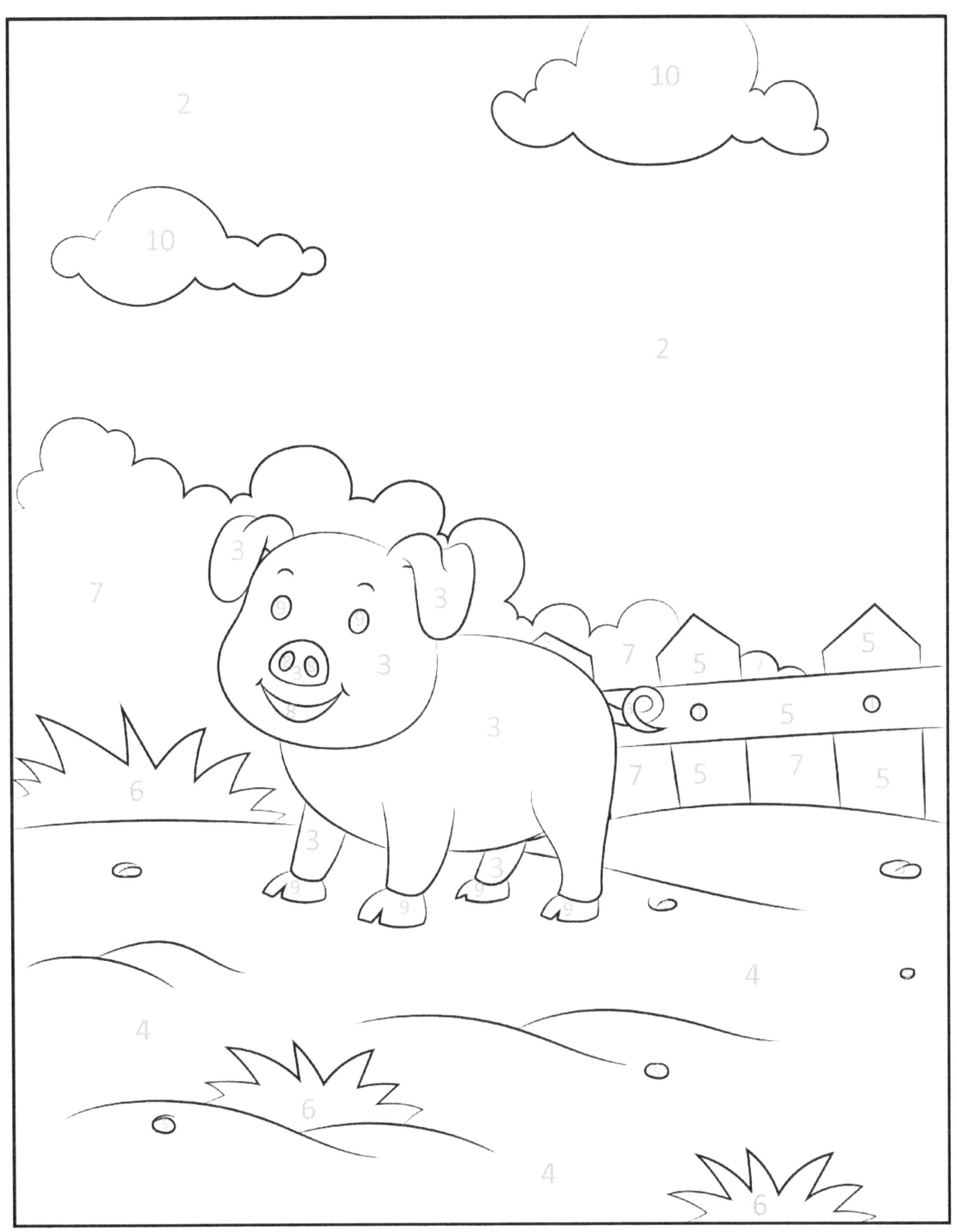

1 – Red	3 – Pink	5 – Brown	7 – Dark Green	9 – Black
2 – Blue	4 – Light Green	6 – Green	8 – Dark Pink	10 – White

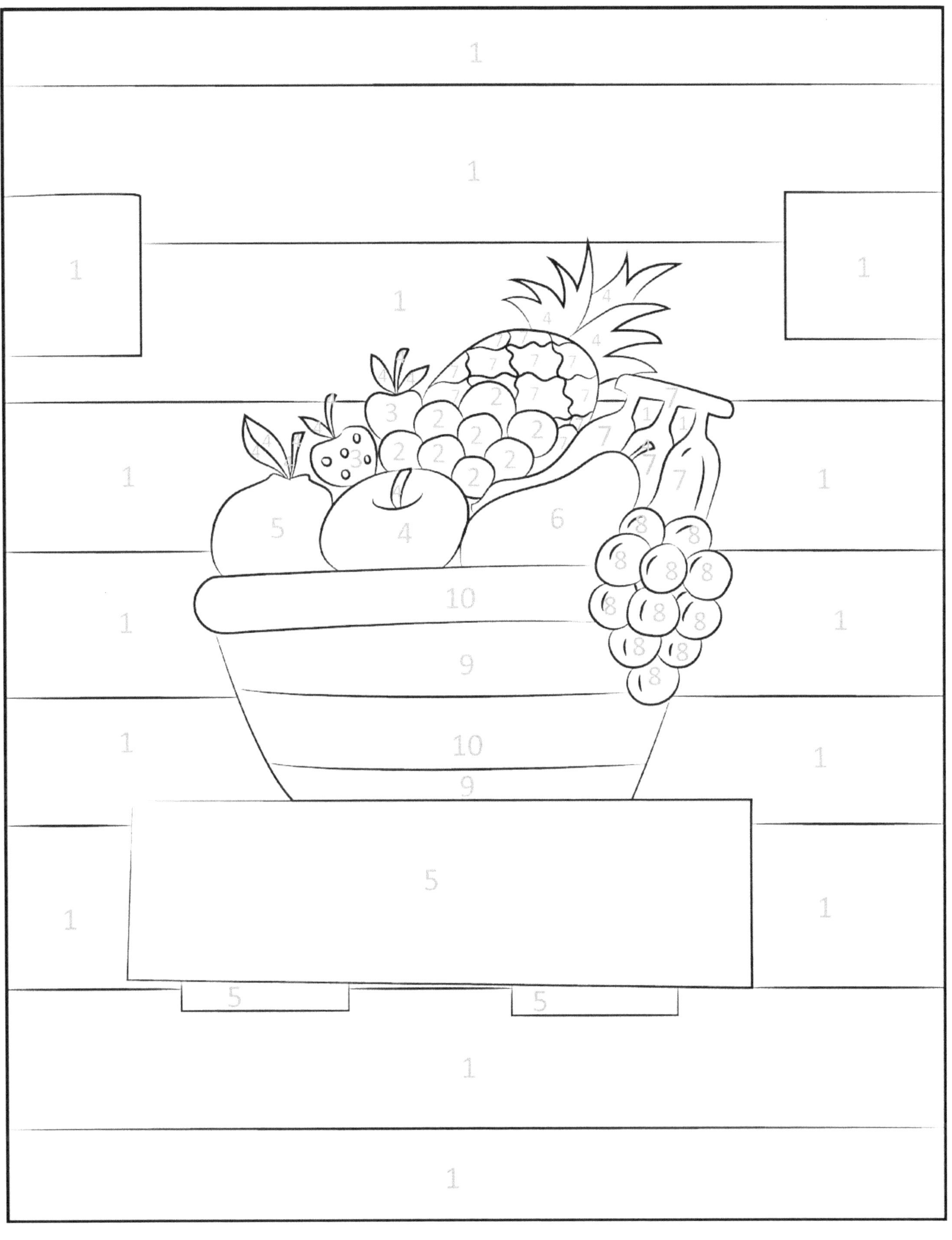

1 – Brown
2 – Purple
3 – Red
4 – Dark Green
5 – Orange
6 – Light Green
7 – Yellow
8 – Green
9 – Black
10 – Pink

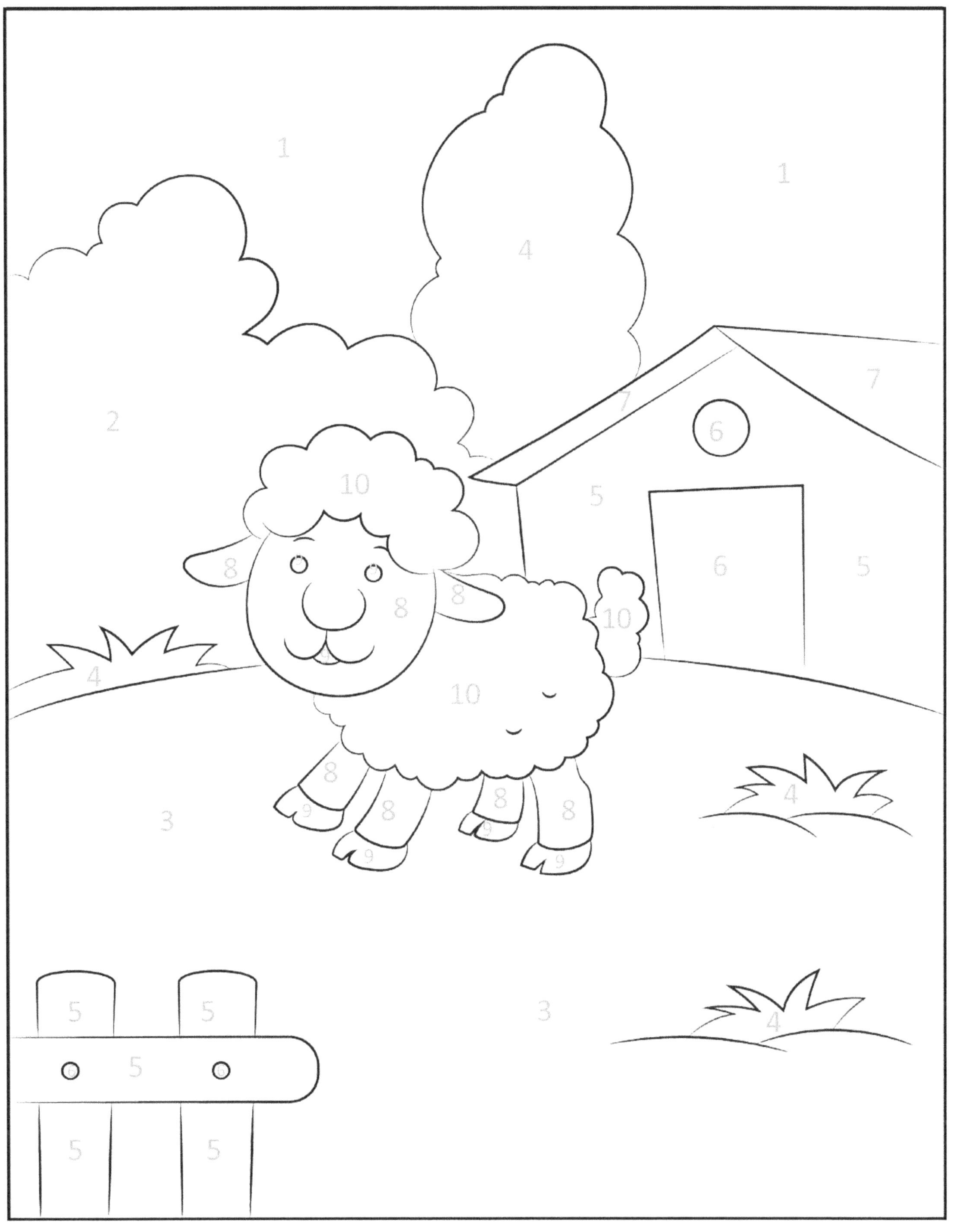

1 – Blue	3 – Light Green	5 – Red	7 – Purple	9 – Black
2 – Green	4 – Dark Green	6 – Yellow	8 – Pink	10 – Grey

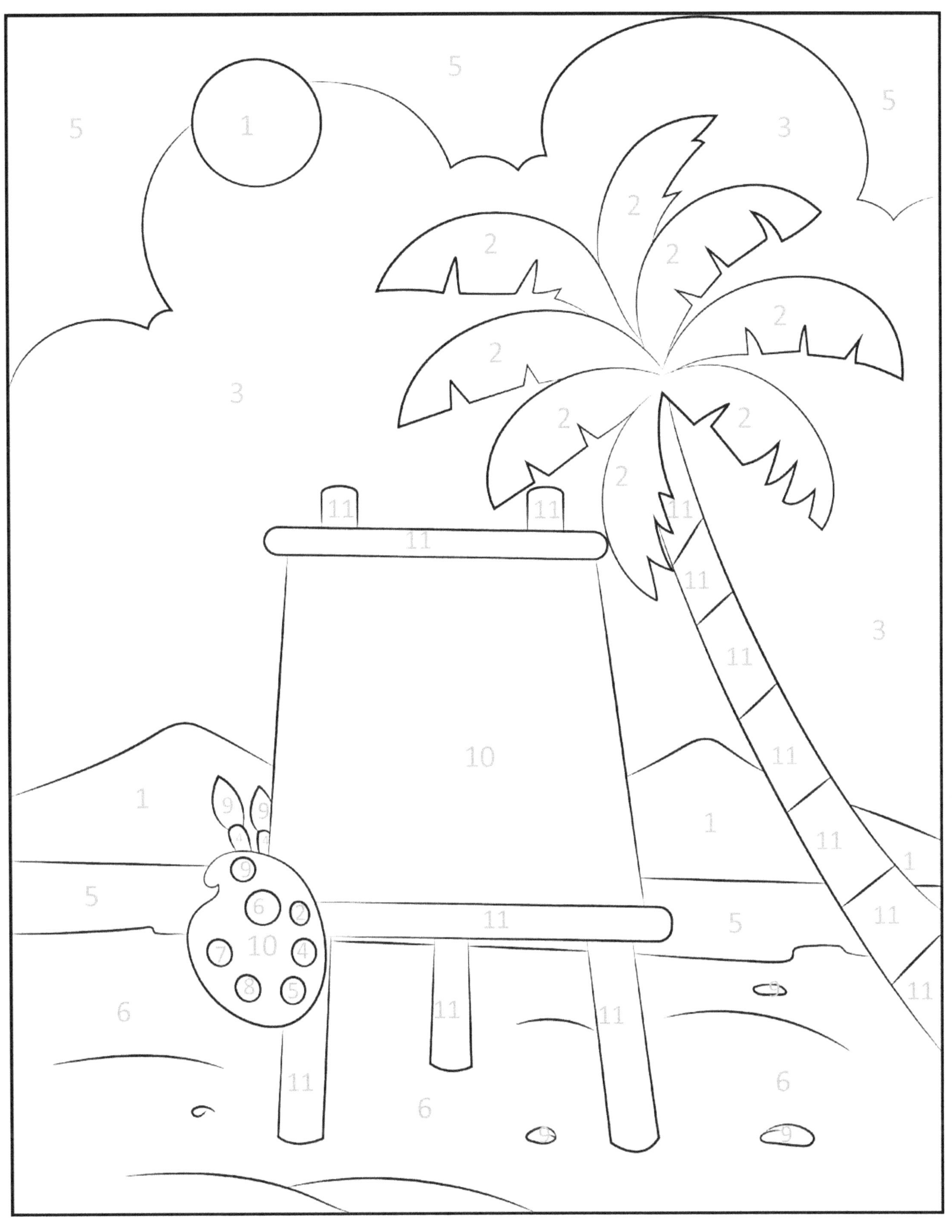

1 – Orange   3 – Light Blue   5 – Blue   7 – Pink   9 – Black   11 – Brown
2 – Dark Green   4 – Red   6 – Yellow   8 – Purple   10 – White

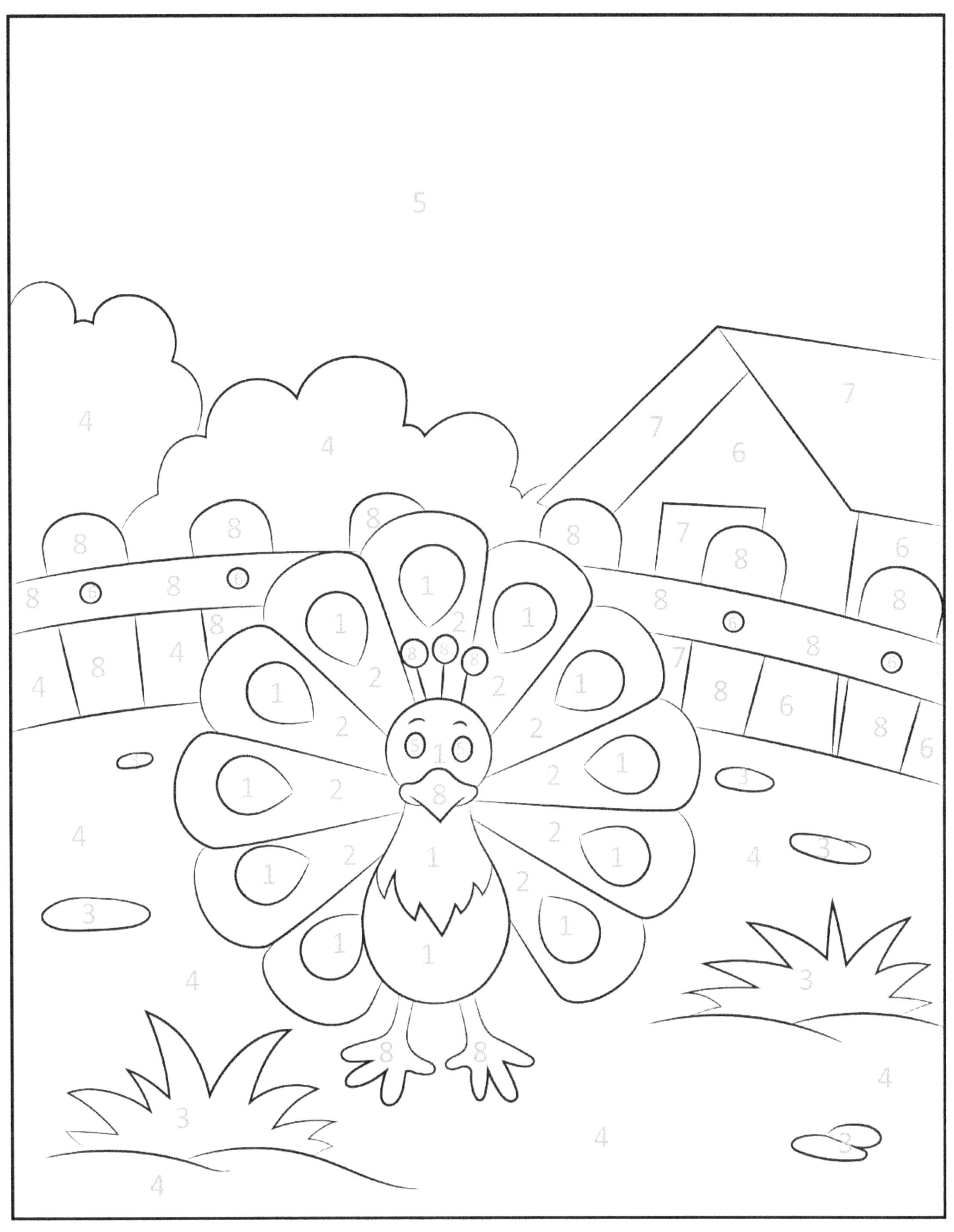

1 – Purple	3 – Light Green	5 – Blue	7 – Orange
2 – Turquoise	4 – Green	6 – Red	8 – Yellow

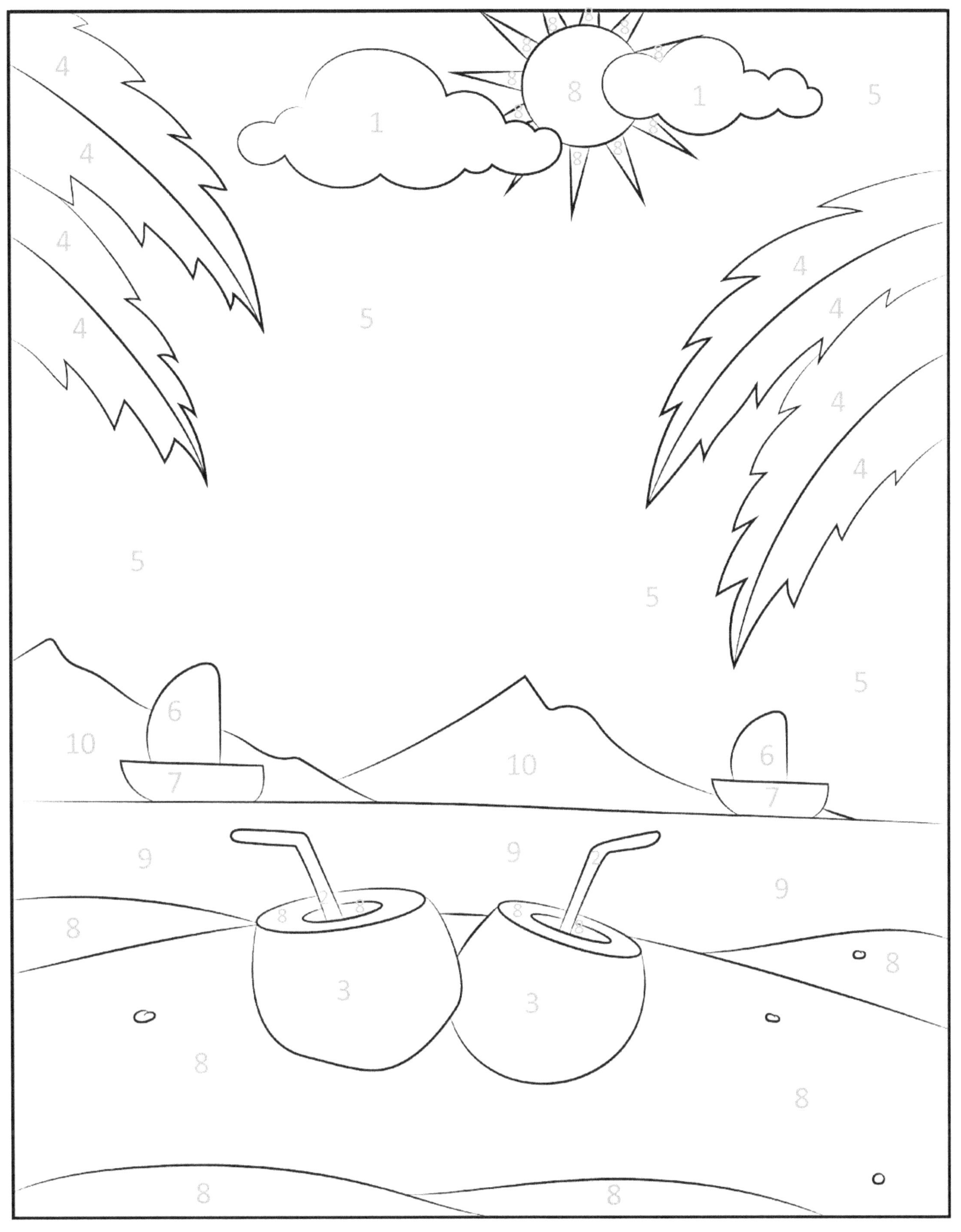

1 – Light Blue	3 – Light Green	5 – Blue	7 – Red	9 – Dark Blue
2 – Green	4 – Dark Green	6 – Pink	8 – Yellow	10 – Orange

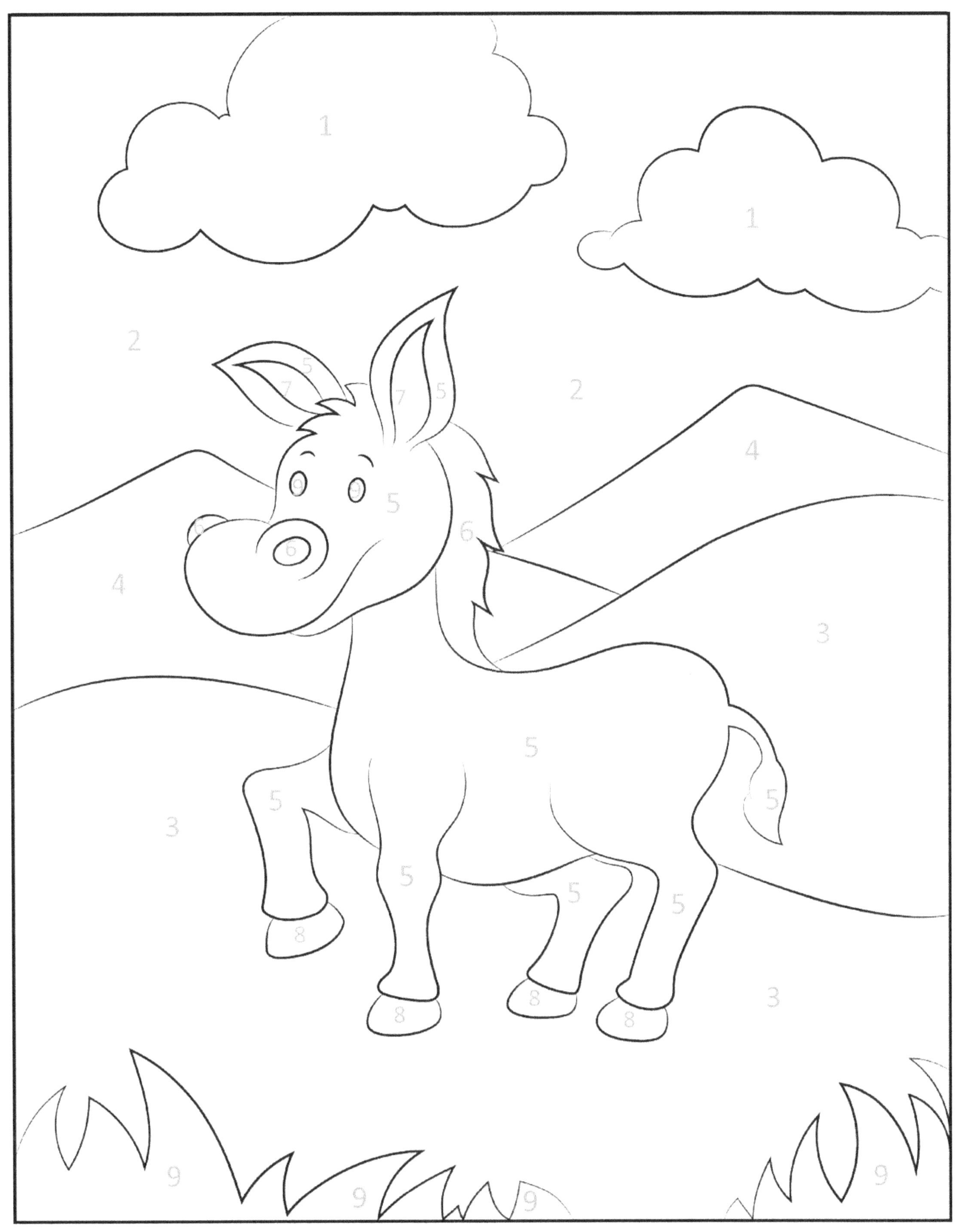

1 – Light Blue   3 – Light Green   5 – Light Brown   7 – Light Pink   9 – Green
2 – Blue   4 – Yellow   6 – Dark Brown   8 – Black

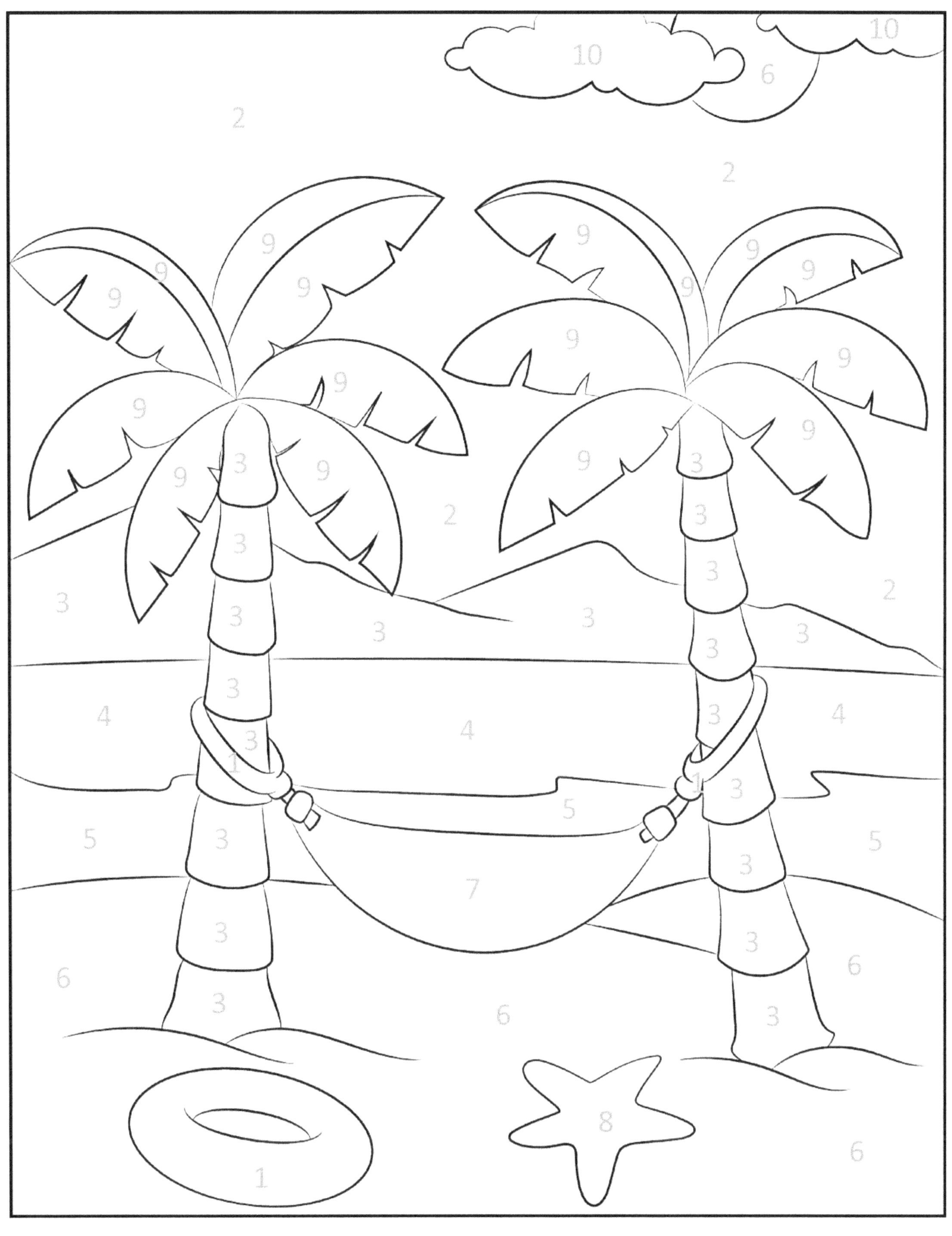

1 – Red
2 – Blue
3 – Dark Brown
4 – Dark Blue
5 – Yellow
6 – Orange
7 – Purple
8 – Dark Yellow
9 – Green
10 – Light Blue

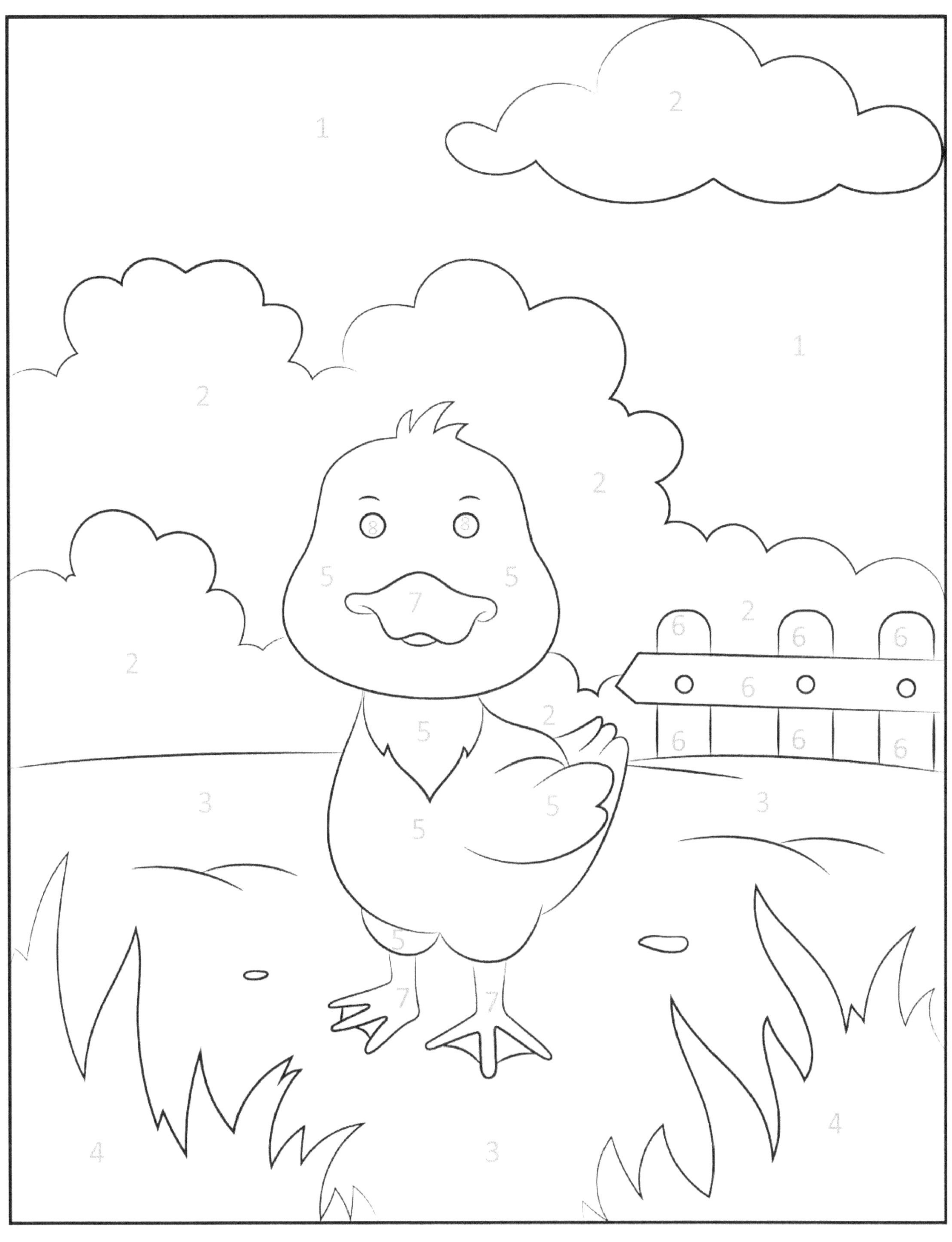

1 – Blue
2 – Light Blue
3 – Green
4 – Dark Green
5 – Yellow
6 – Orange
7 – Red
8 – Black

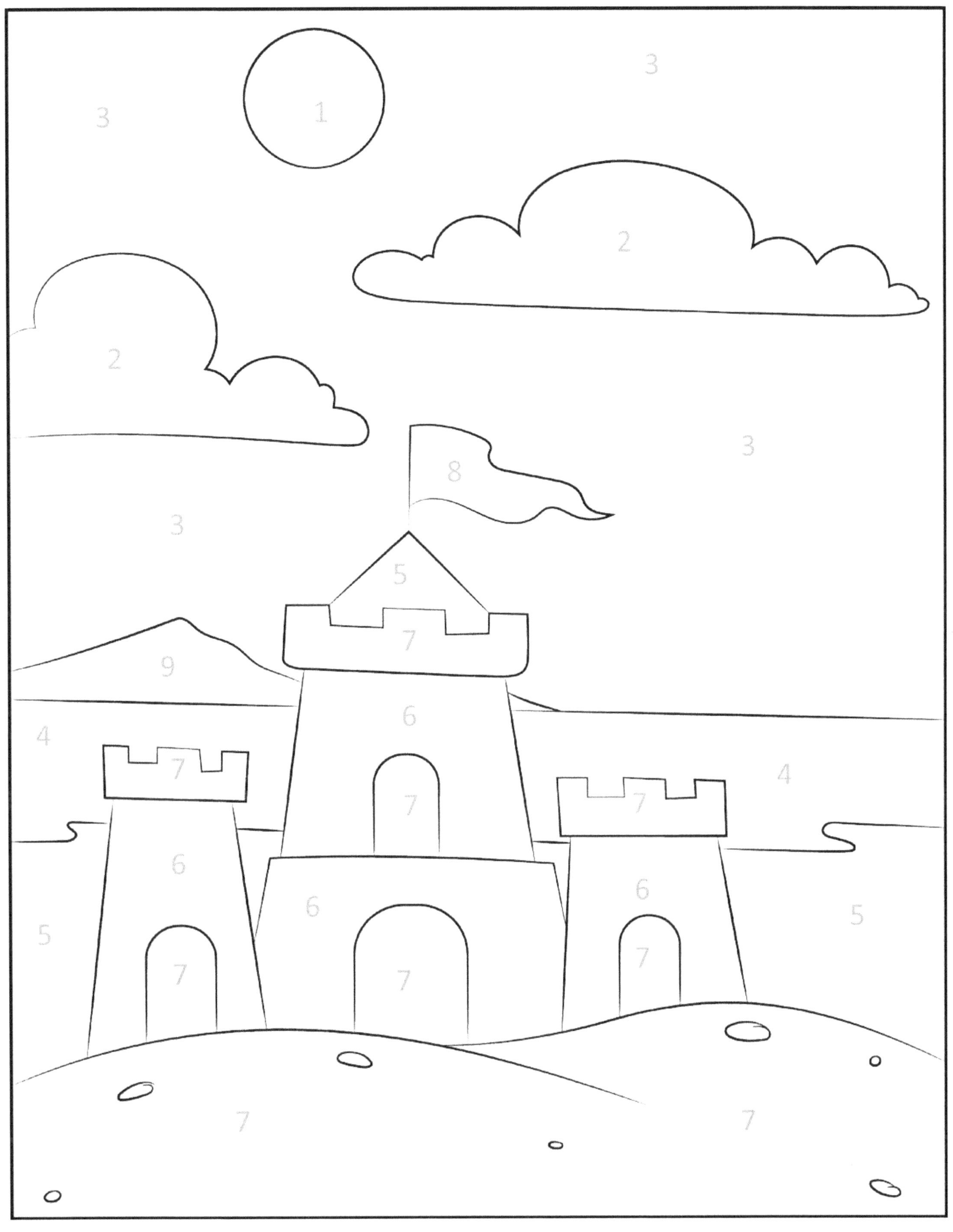

1 – Yellow   3 – Blue   5 – Yellow   7 – Orange   9 – Dark Green
2 – Light Blue   4 – Dark Blue   6 – Light Brown   8 – Red

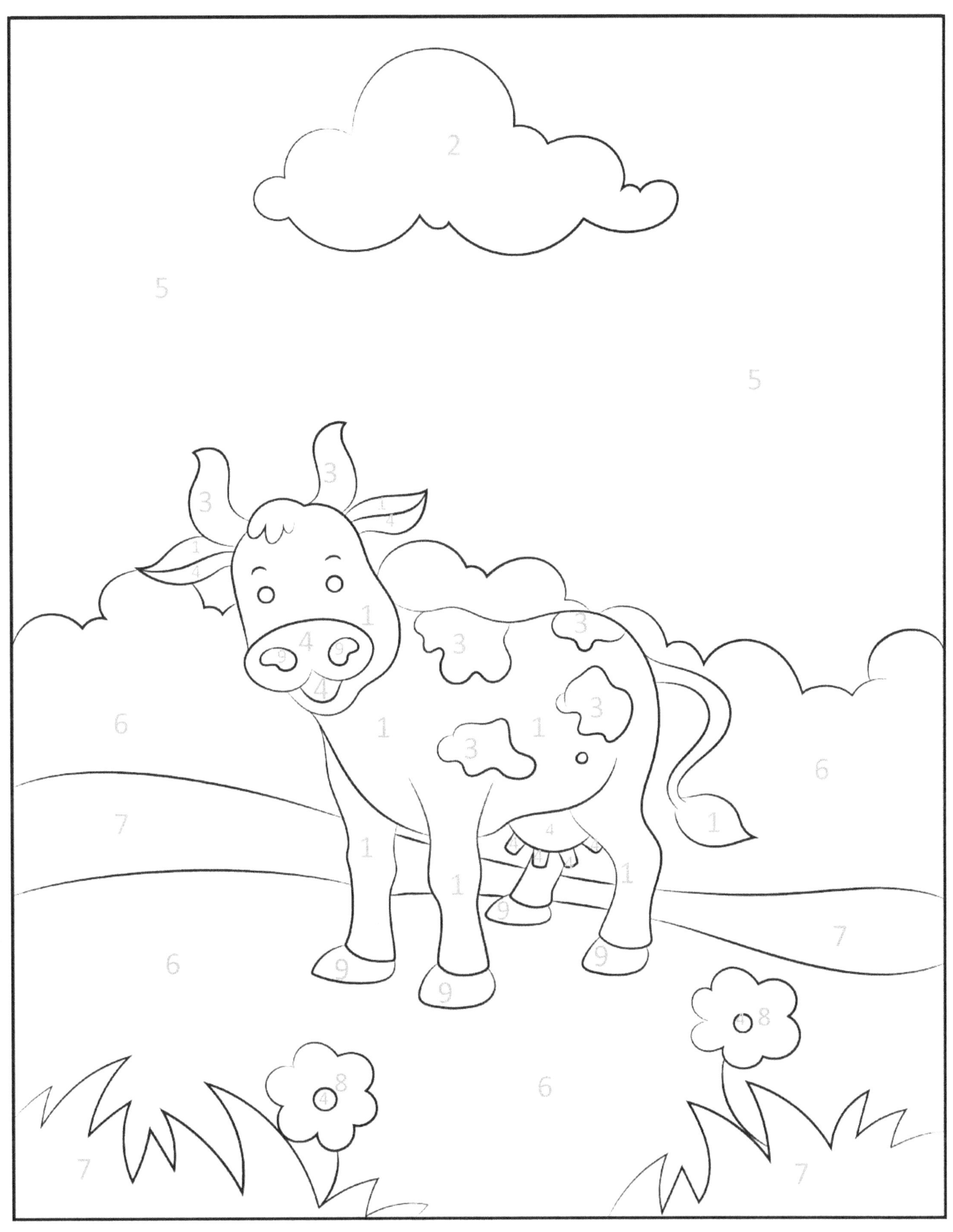

1 – White   3 – Brown   5 – Blue   7 – Dark Green   9 – Black
2 – Light Blue   4 – Pink   6 – Green   8 – Yellow

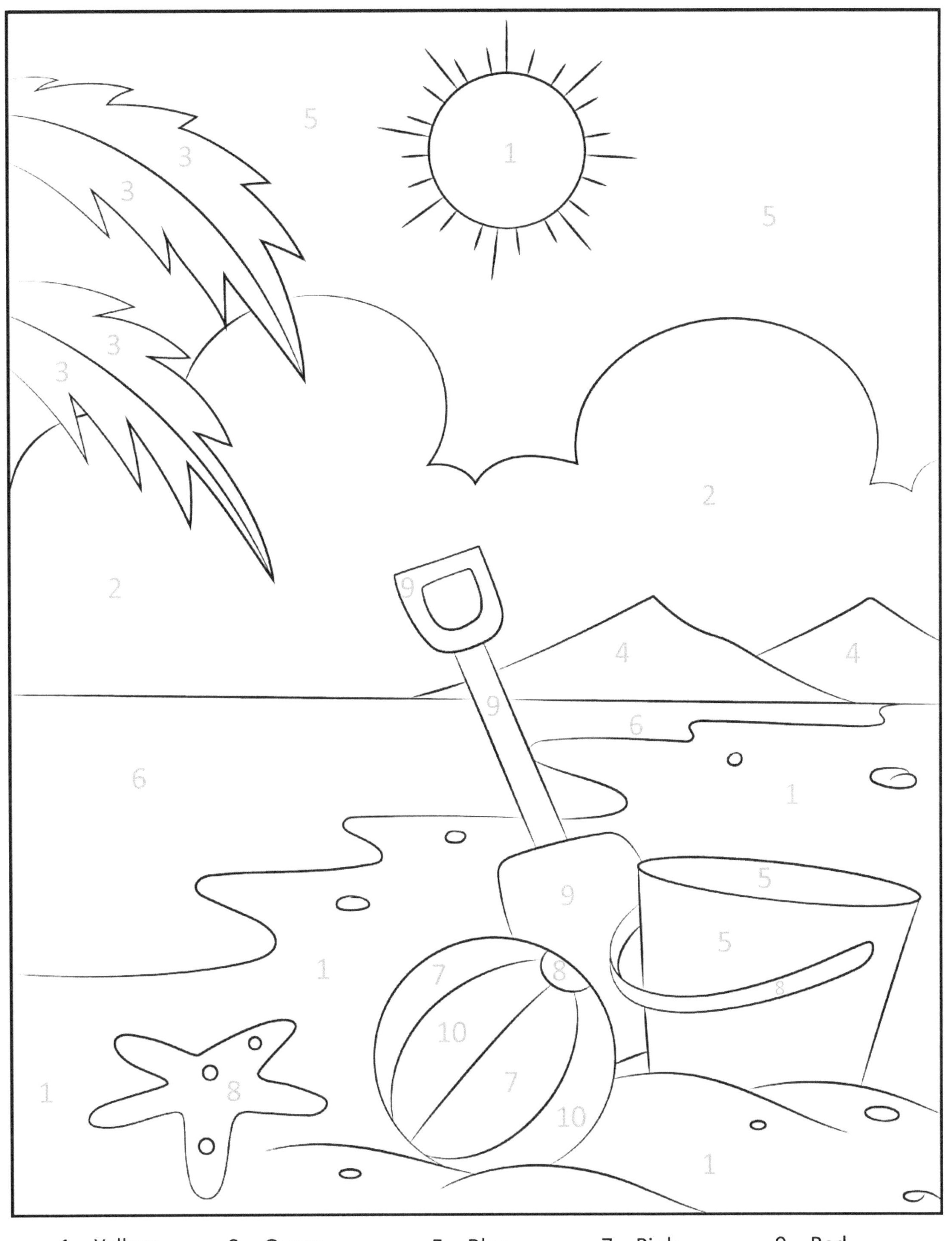

1 – Yellow
2 – White
3 – Green
4 – Dark Green
5 – Blue
6 – Dark Blue
7 – Pink
8 – Orange
9 – Red
10 – Purple

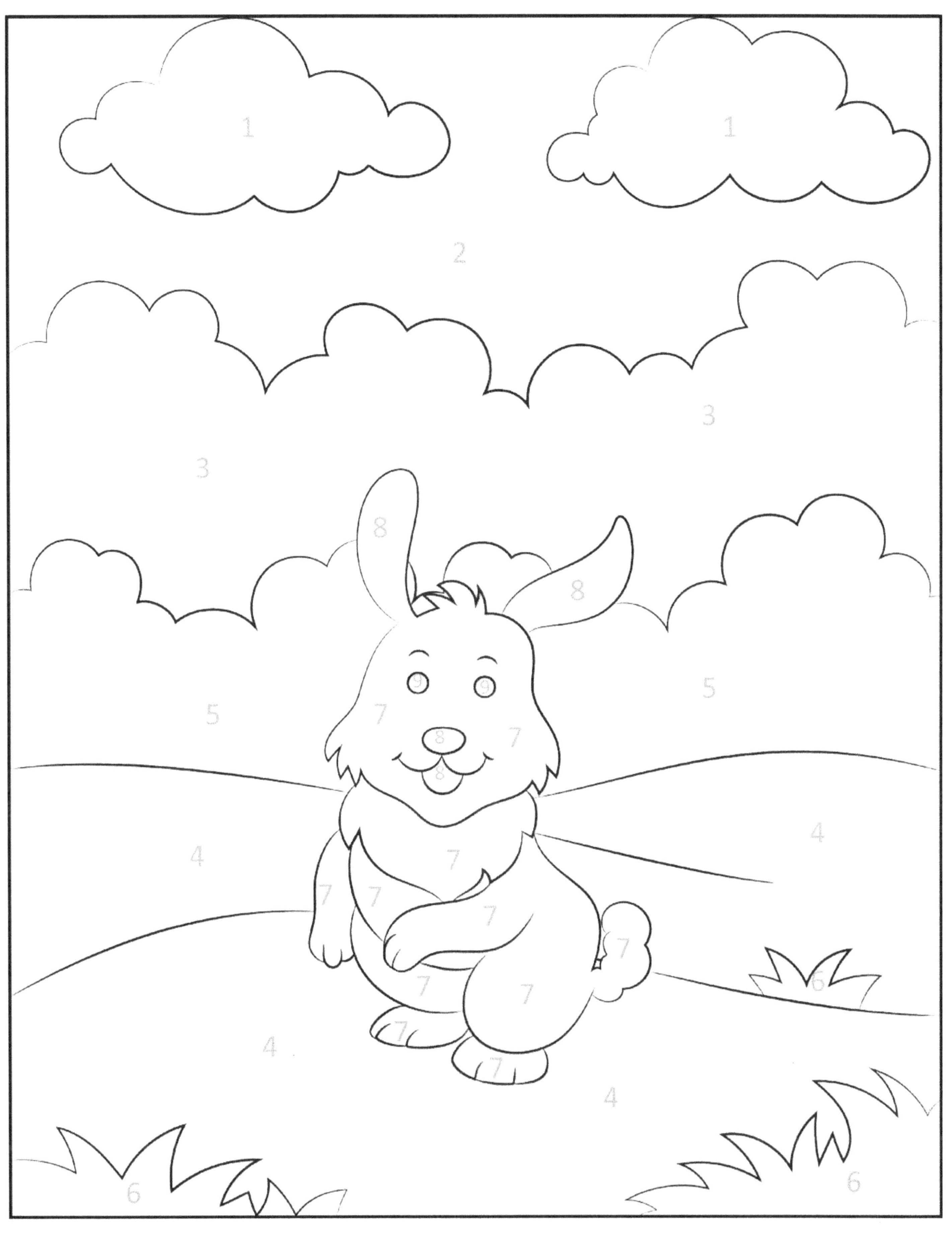

1 – White   3 – Blue   5 – Yellow   7 – Grey   9 – Black
2 – Light Blue   4 – Green   6 – Orange   8 – Pink

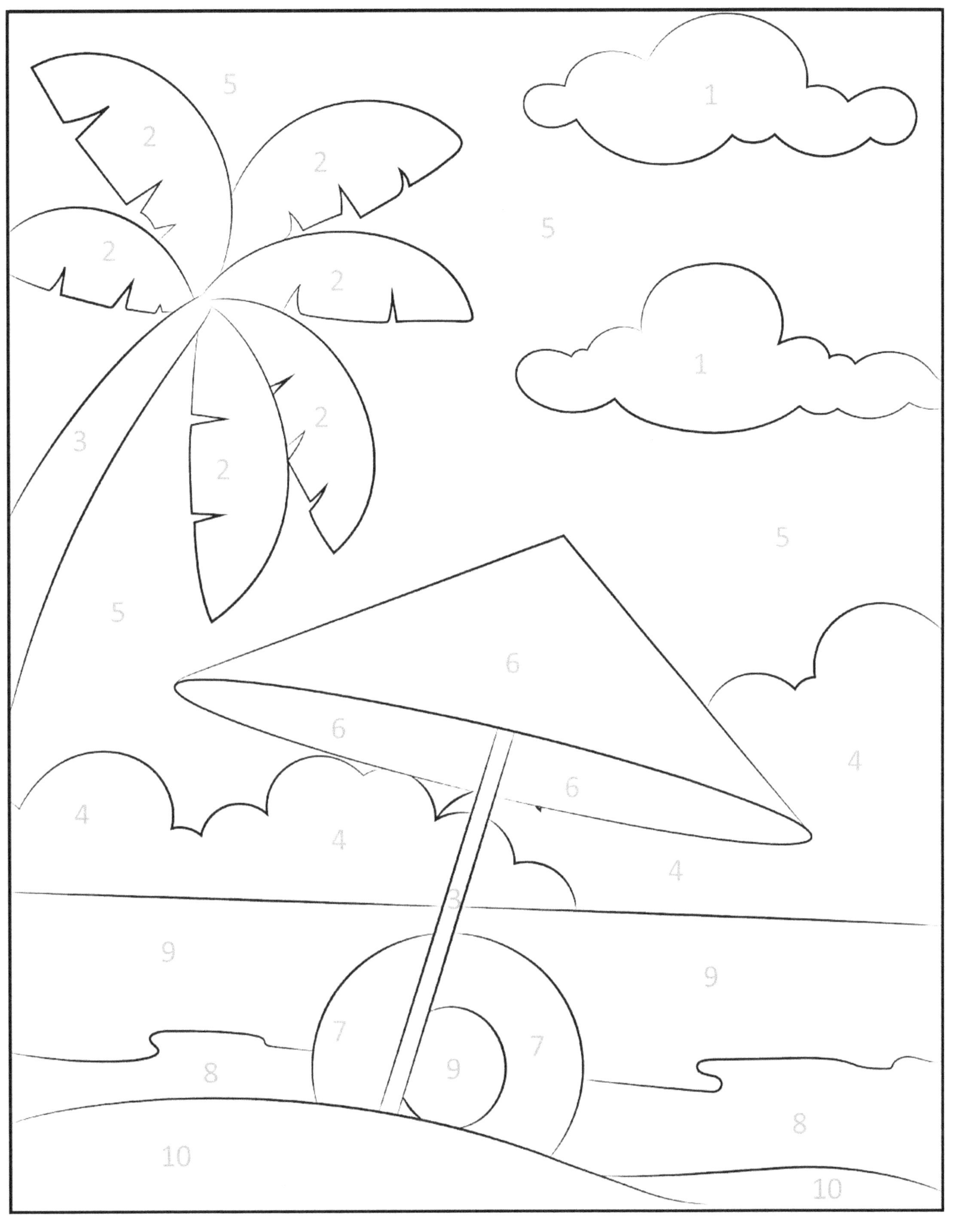

1 – Grey
2 – Green
3 – Brown
4 – Dark Green
5 – Blue
6 – Red
7 – Purple
8 – Light Brown
9 – Aqua
10 – Yellow

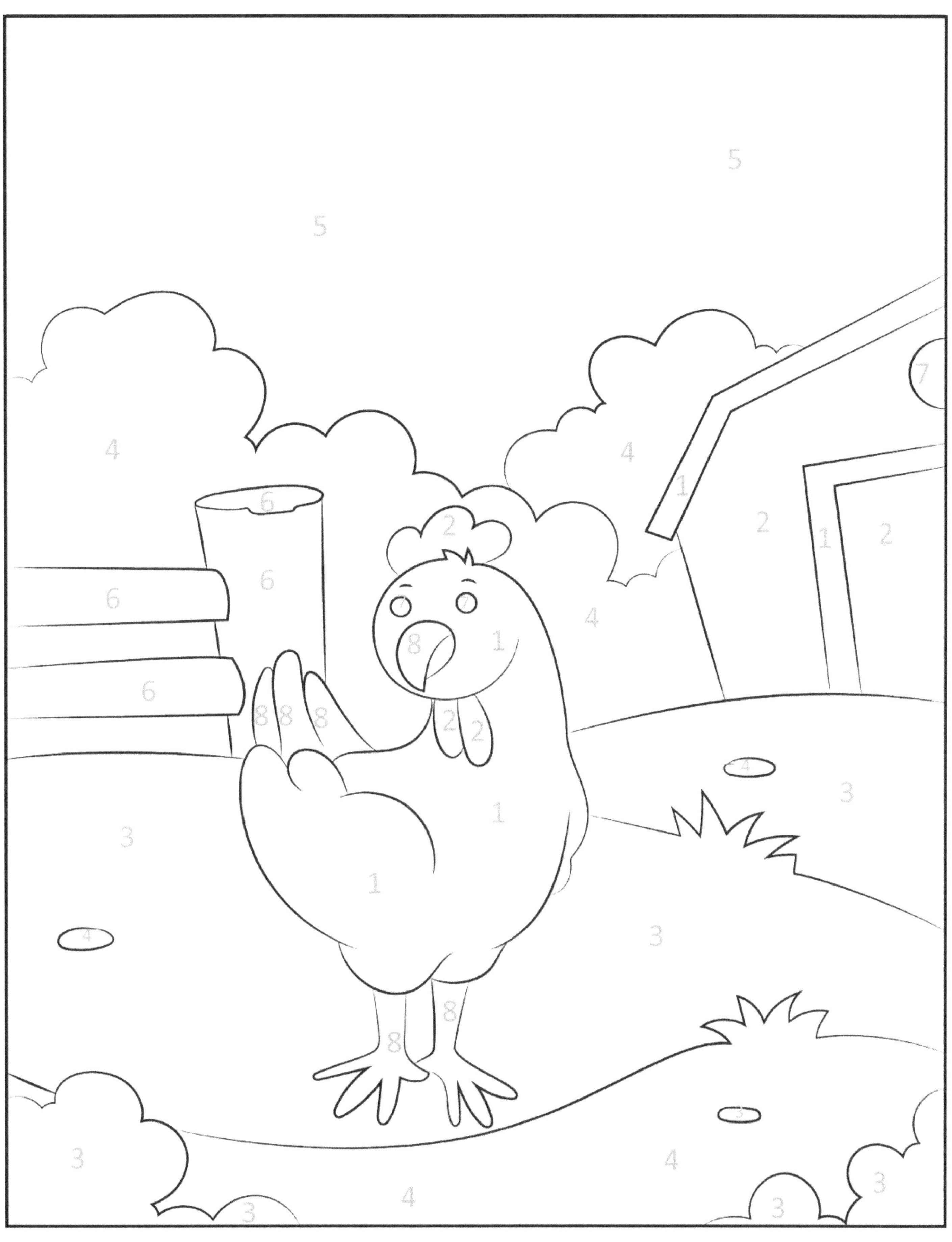

1 – Yellow	3 – Green	5 – Blue	7 – Black
2 – Red	4 – Dark Green	6 – Brown	8 – Orange

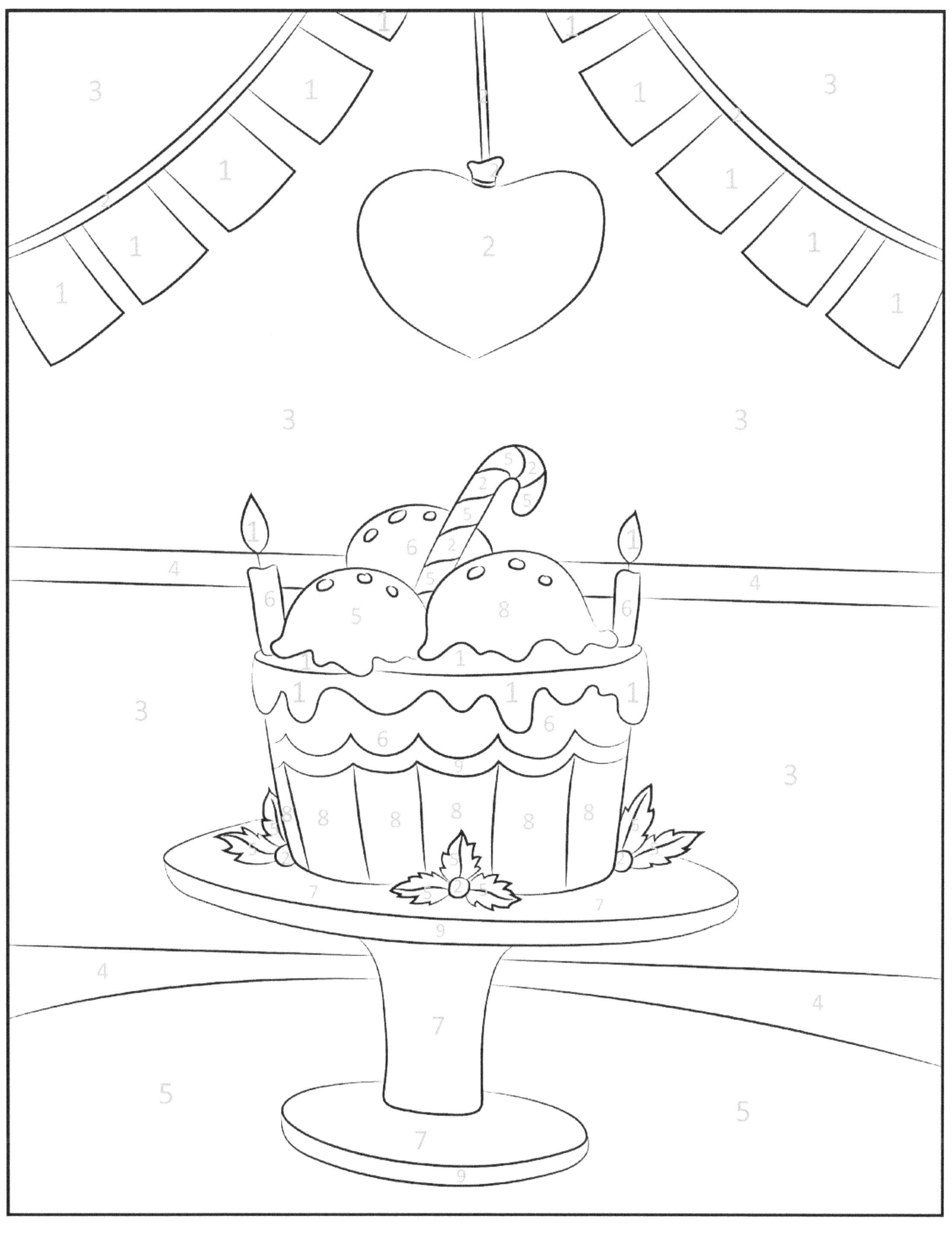

1 – Yellow   3 – Blue   5 – Green   7 – Black   9 – White
2 – Red   4 – Orange   6 – Pink   8 – Purple

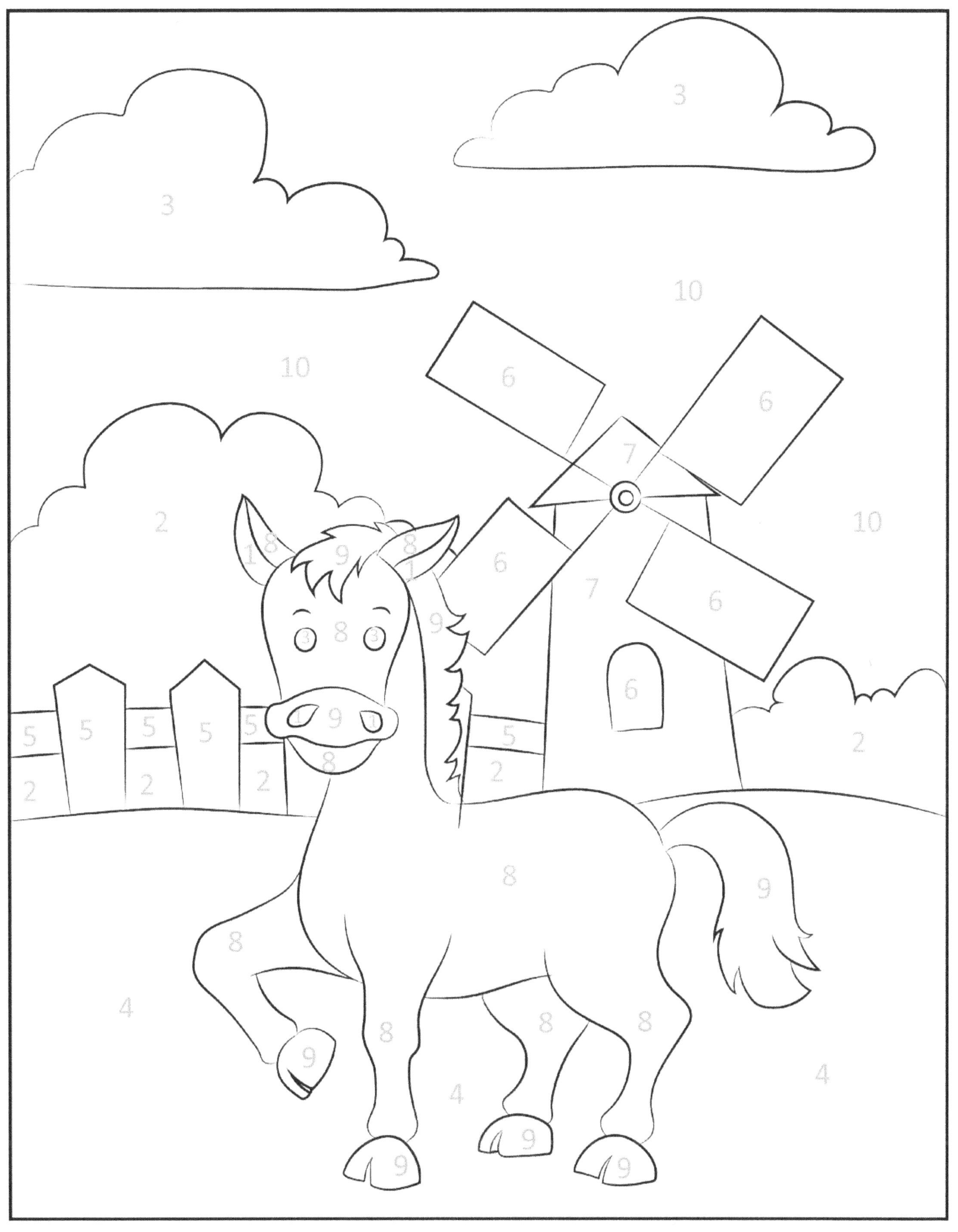

1 – Pink	3 – Light Blue	5 – Yellow	7 – Orange	9 – Black
2 – Dark Green	4 – Green	6 – Red	8 – Light Brown	10 – Blue

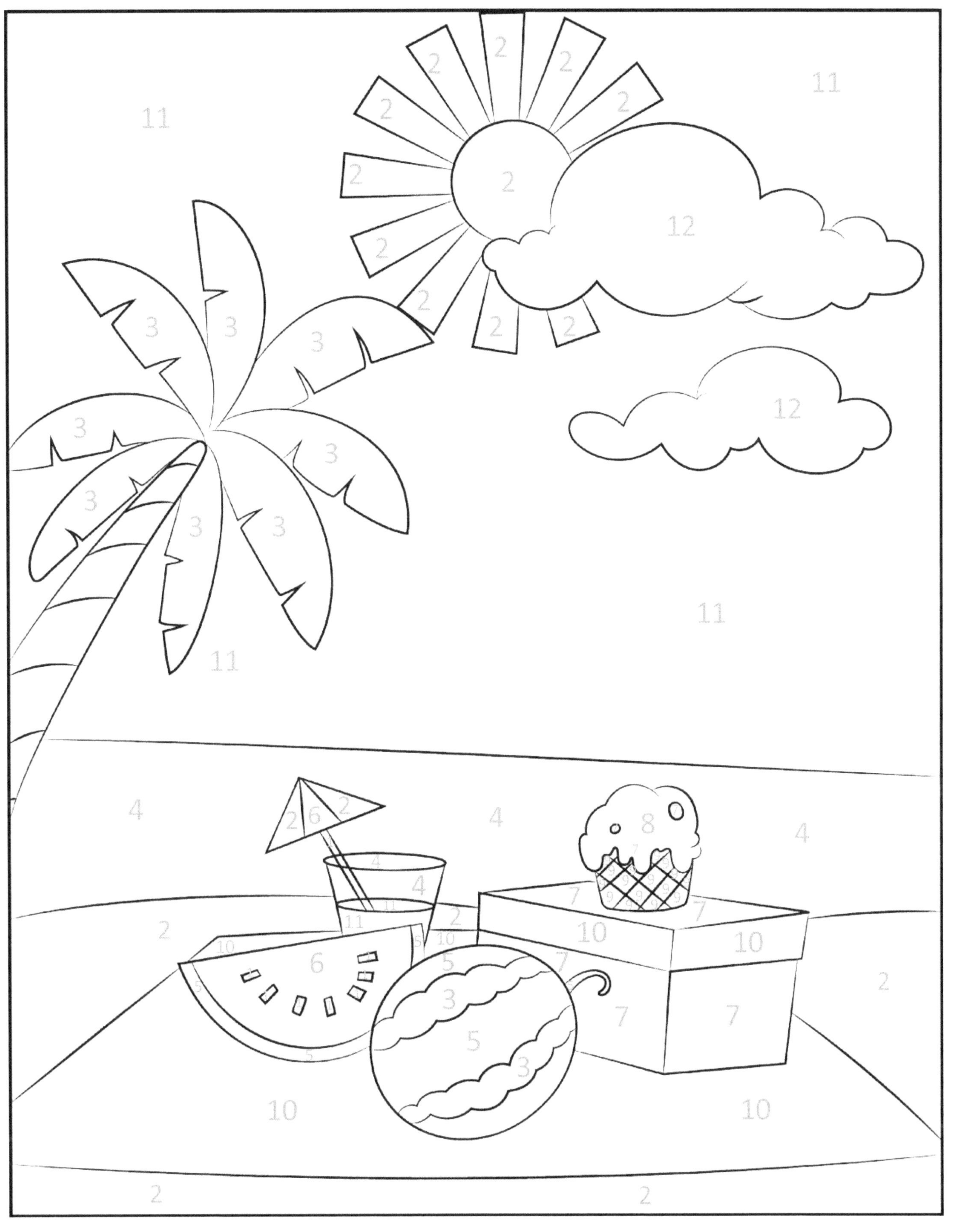

1 – Black
2 – Yellow
3 – Green
4 – Turquoise
5 – Dark Green
6 – Red
7 – Pink
8 – White
9 – Orange
10 – Purple
11 – Blue
12 – Light Blue

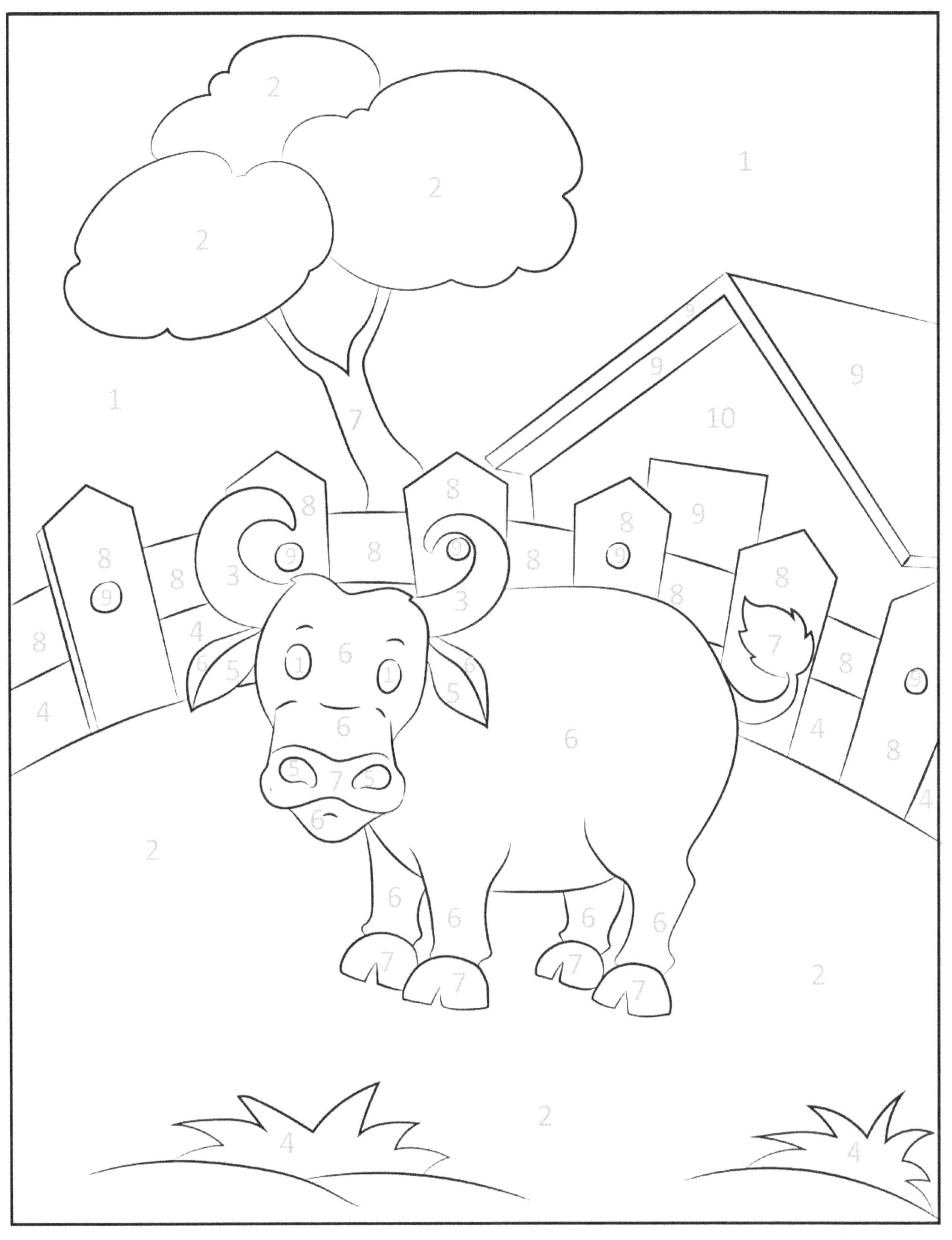

1 – Light Blue   3 – Light Brown   5 – Pink   7 – Dark Brown   9 – Red
2 – Green   4 – Dark Green   6 – Brown   8 – Yellow   10 – Orange

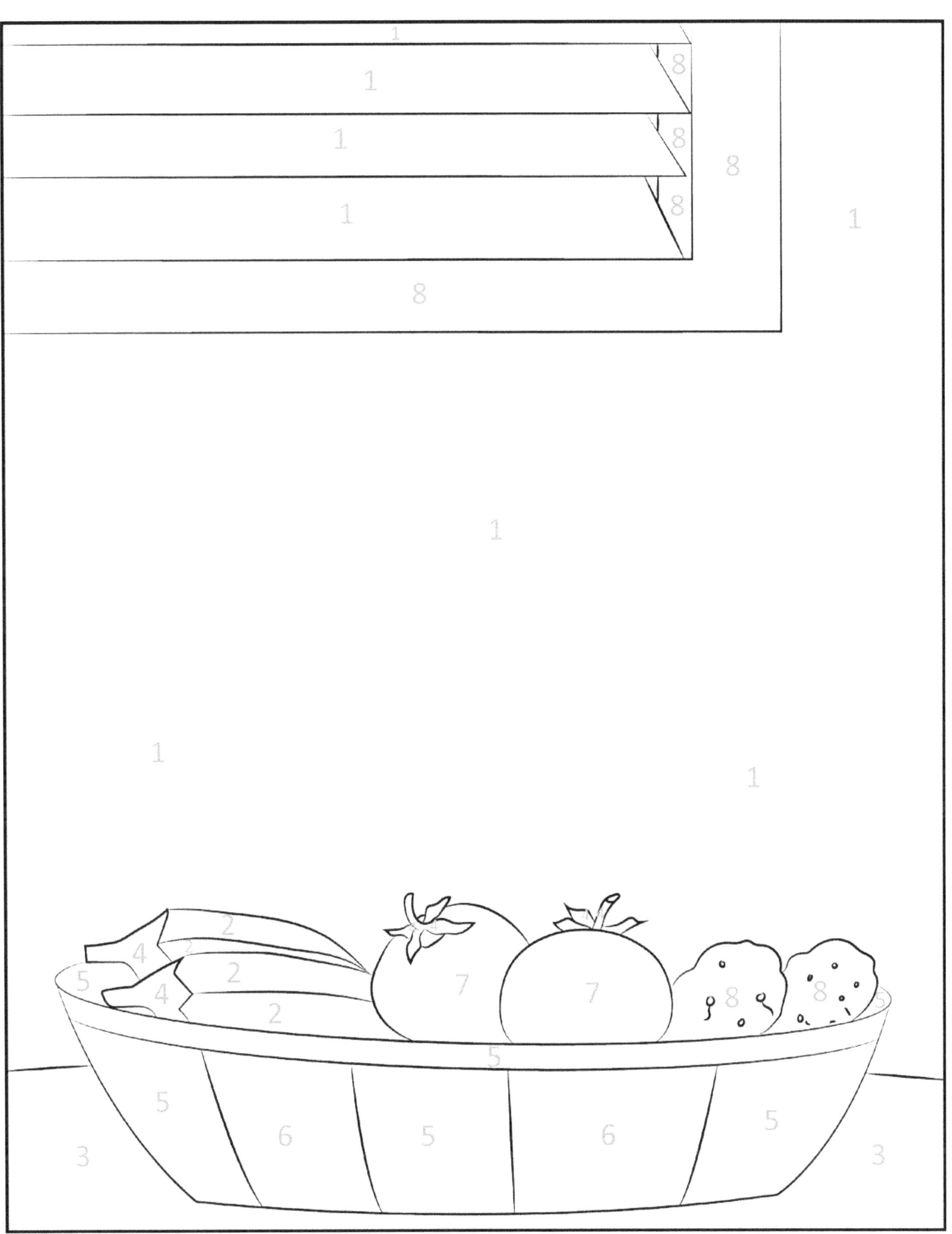

1 – Light Brown
2 – Green
3 – Light Green
4 – Dark Green
5 – Blue
6 – Dark Blue
7 – Red
8 – Dark Brown

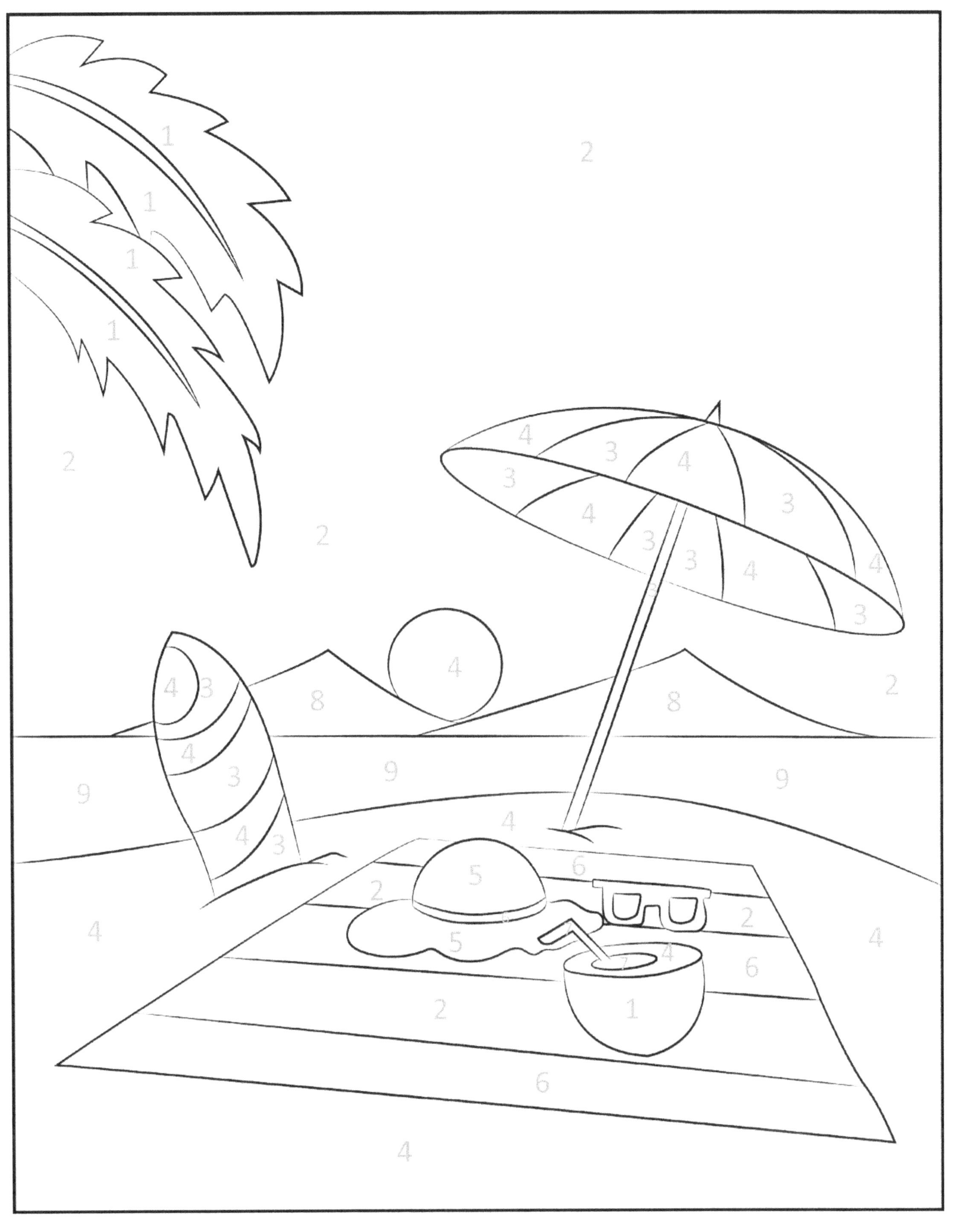

1 – Green
2 – Blue
3 – Red
4 – Yellow
5 – Pink
6 – Purple
7 – White
8 – Dark Green
9 – Dark Blue

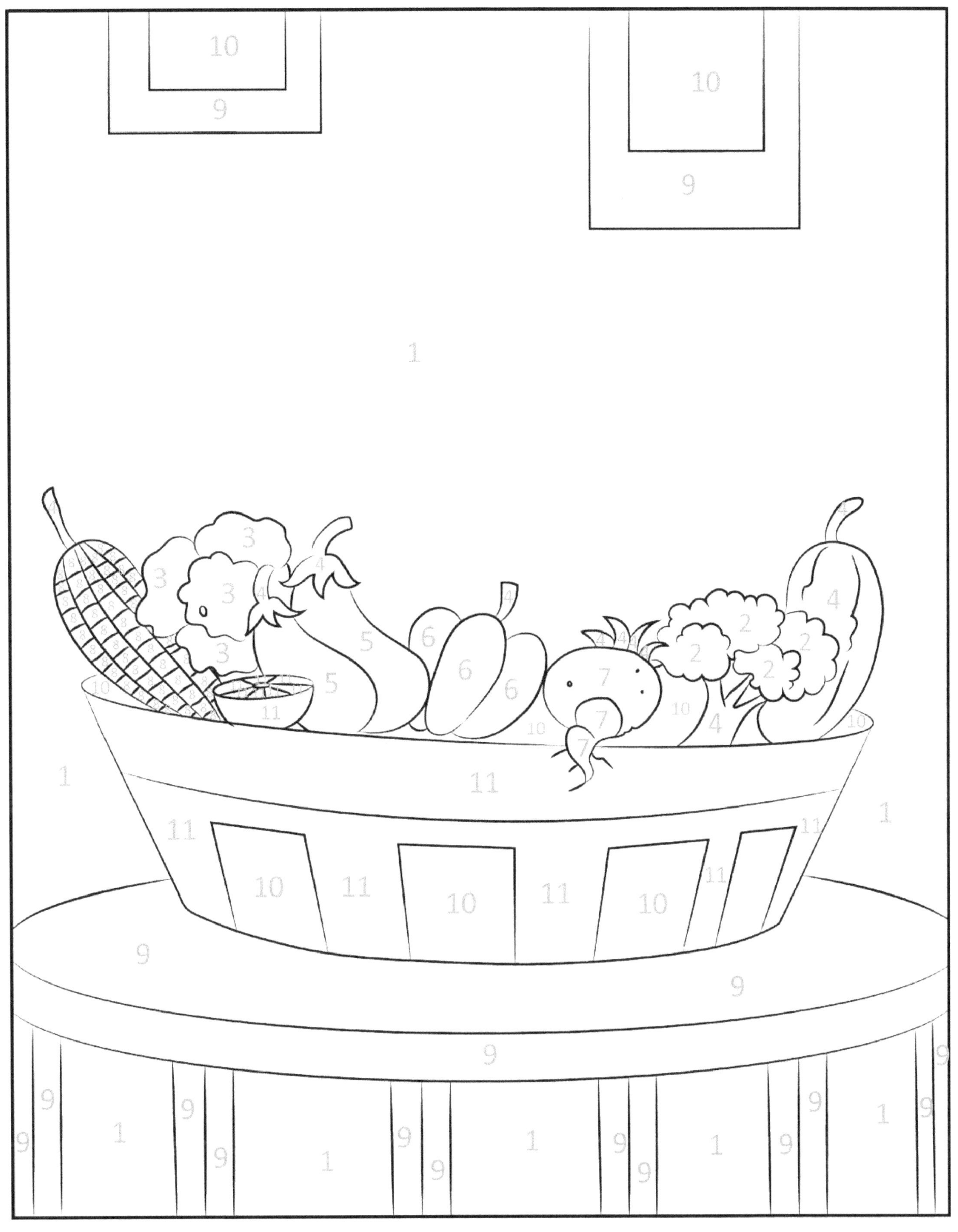

1 – Light Pink   3 – Light Green   5 – Purple   7 – Light Brown   9 – Black   11 – Orange
2 – Green   4 – Dark Green   6 – Red   8 – Yellow   10 – Grey

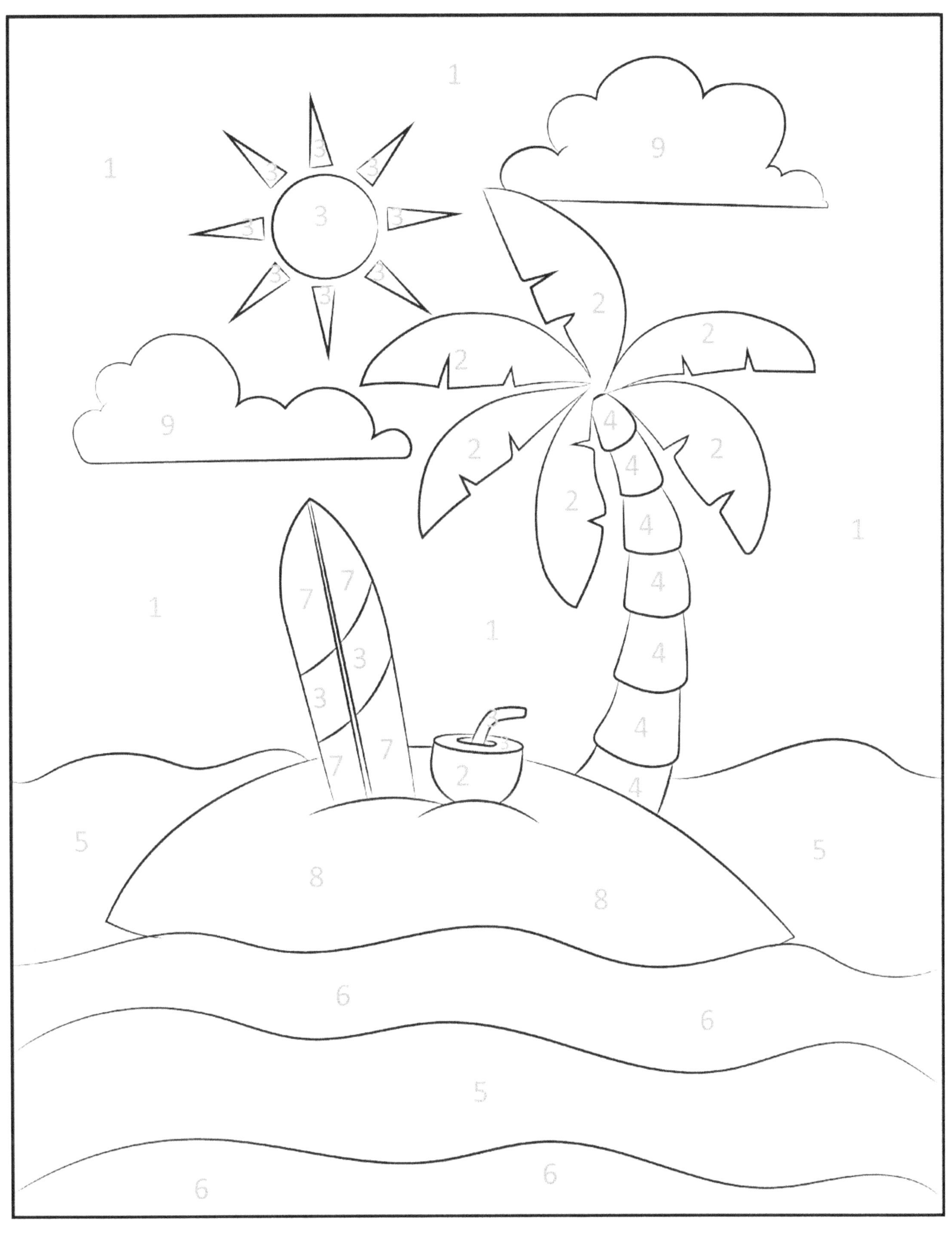

1 – Light Blue	3 – Yellow	5 – Blue	7 – Pink	9 – Light Grey
2 – Green	4 – Brown	6 – Dark Blue	8 – Orange	

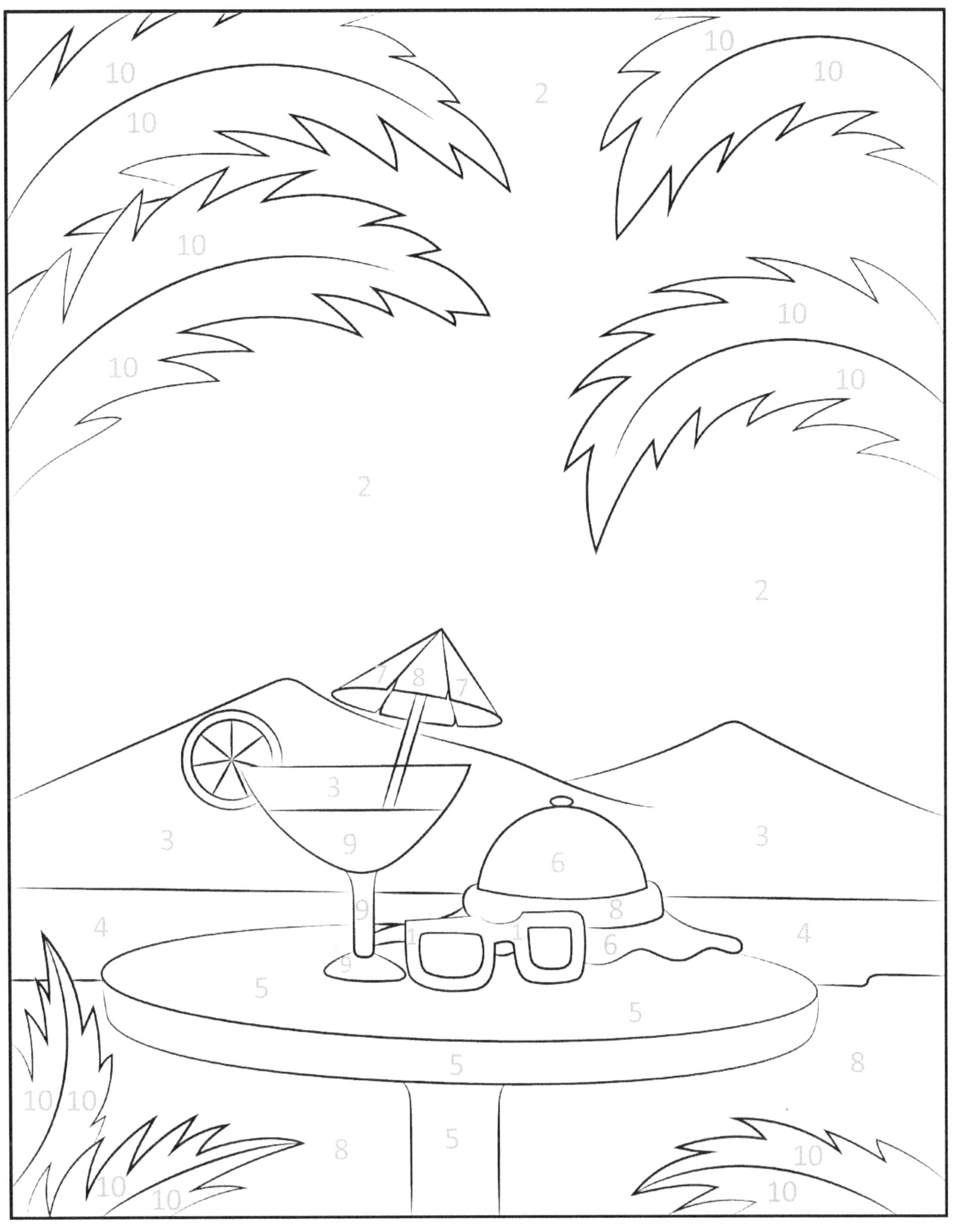

1 – Red
2 – Blue
3 – Light Brown
4 – Dark Blue
5 – Black
6 – Pink
7 – Purple
8 – Yellow
9 – Aqua
10 – Green

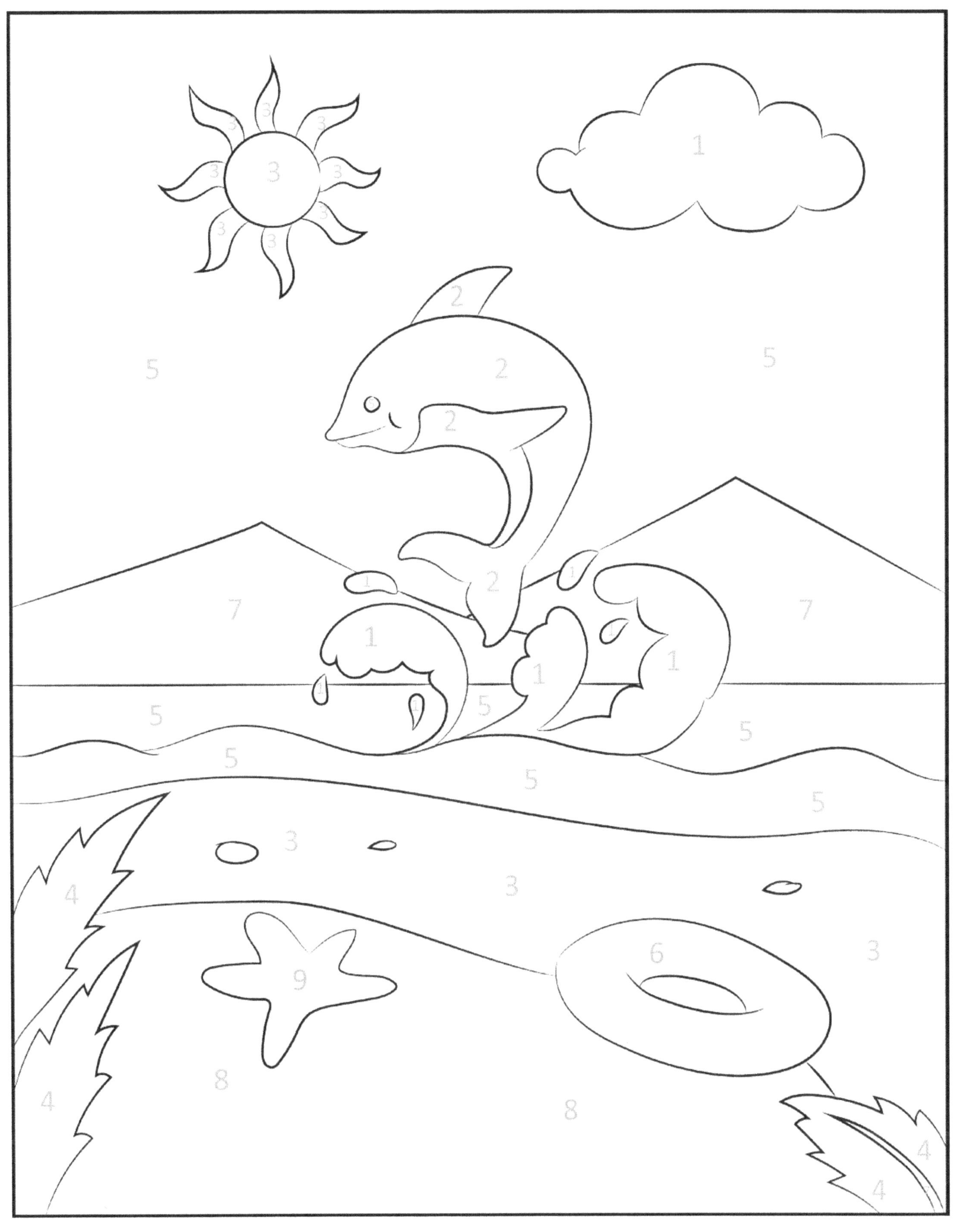

1 – Light Blue	3 – Yellow	5 – Blue	7 – Dark Green	9 – Purple
2 – Grey	4 – Green	6 – Pink	8 – Orange	

Thank you for your purchase ☺

If you enjoyed this book, I'd love it if you would please share your thoughts by leaving a review!

As a Creative Designer, I would like to invite you to check-out my other creations that you may find helpful in your life and at home.

Find me here on Etsy to Print at Home:

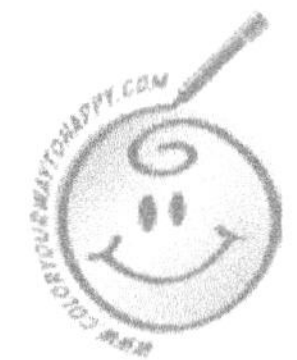

Color Your Way To Happy
Print at home coloring books for adults and kids to color for fun, relaxation and stress relief.
http://www.ColorYourWayToHappy.etsy.com

Organized Life and Home
Beautiful and practical PDF Digital Download printables, to print at home to organize your Life and Home.
http://www.OrganizedLifeandHome.etsy.com

Find me here on Amazon:

Nerine Martin/Color Your Way to Happy
Coloring books for adults and kids.
www.ColorYourWayToHappy.com

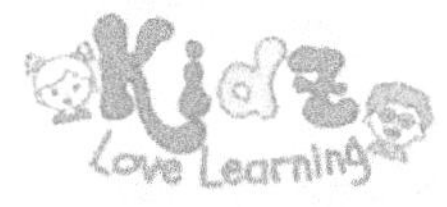

Kidz Love Learning
Activity and learning books for kids and home schooling.
www.KidzLoveLearning.com

Organized Life and Home
Planners, journals and logbooks to keep you organized.
www.OrganizedLifeandHome.com